Your Guide to Smooth Sailing With Transformational Tales

My daughter is shy and doesn't like to talk in class.

Try The Frog Story

I seem to be angry a lot.

The Bear or The Raccoon Story.

My anxiety is keeping me from sleeping.

The Bunny Story is good for that.

Someone I love is getting a knee replacement.

The Critter helps acceptance

Our relationship is quite bad.

You both might want to read The Magic Bridges.

SAILING THROUGH THE RAINBOW

Transformational Tales

Mary Jayne Collins, Ph.D.

ATLATL Publishing
611 Hampshire Rd. #530
Westlake Village, CA 91361
www.atlatlpublishing.com

Atlatl Publishing, Westlake Village, CA 91361

Please visit our Website: www.atlatlpublishing.com

Printed in the United States of America.

07 08 09 10 11 12 13 14 5 4 3 2 1

Library of Congress Control Number: 2007924160

Collins, Mary Jayne.
Sailing Through the Rainbow: Transformational Tales

ISBN 978-0-9793366-0-7

To

My husband David,
And to my children,
grandchildren, great-grandchildren,
and friends who fill my life with
meaning and blessings.

Contents

How To Read This Book

THESE stories bypass your critical mind and talk to the *you* behind your conscious thoughts. That is where you access the wise and profound part of your mind. Your mind can choose unique and personally meaningful connections, changing you at a subconscious level. That is why the stories are called *transformational.* These stories are different because the specific image metaphors were purposely chosen, and then the story was woven around them.

Transformational tales can do much to help us deal with life. Valuable attributes can be discovered and strengthened, such as wisdom, courage, integrity, trust, or compassion. These stories are designed for specific purposes. They can help reduce fear and anxiety, can help us to learn to deal with anger. They can help us trust our inner guidance, increase courage and speed up our natural ability to heal. Stories can assist us in adjusting to necessary, though unwanted events, can help us not give up. These tales can increase hope, can help us become more open to new ideas, attitudes and experiences, accept change and can help us get unstuck. Stories can help reduce our feelings of isolation, thereby helping us to feel our connection to each other and the Creator. They can increase creativity, reduce conflicts, increase teamwork, help us increase our insight and trust our intuition. Summaries at the end of each story discuss some of the issues they may address.

If you are reading the story to someone else, try to help that person to relax and keep him or her free of distractions. Suggest that your listener float along with the story, seeing his own images. There is no need to "make sense" or analyze the stories because much change can be effected by those deeper parts of us that are not conscious. The stories are great for reducing stress. Just use a soft relaxed voice.

If you read the story yourself, try to sink into the story and the images, sounds, smells or feelings that it evokes. These stories are not only for children. Most of them were written for adults. There is a part of us that responds, no matter what our age.

Enjoy.

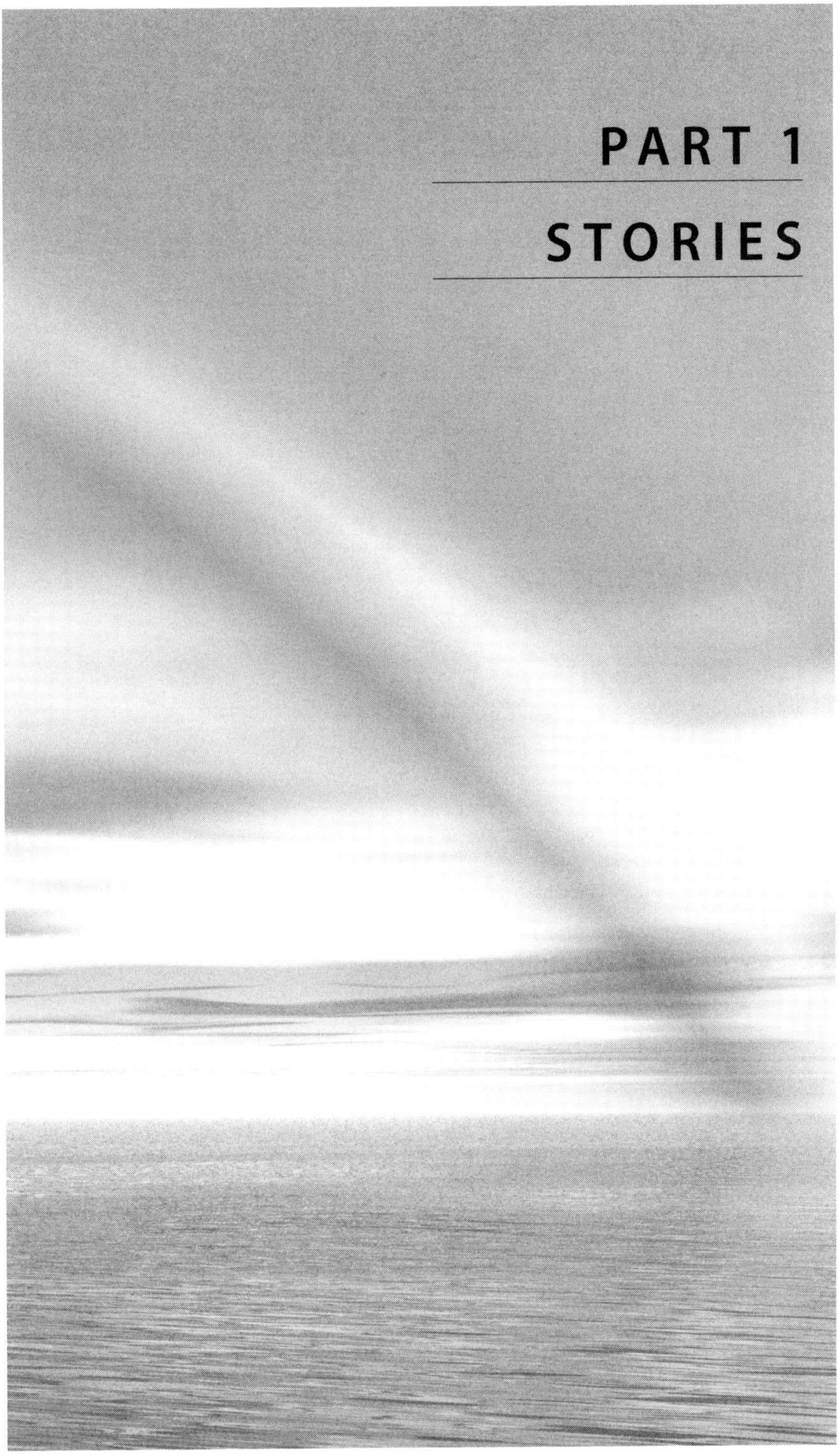

PART 1

STORIES

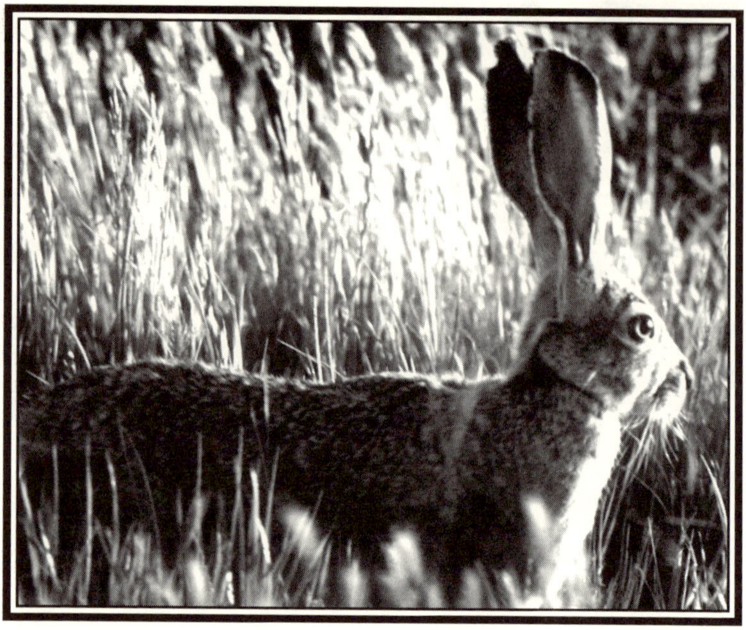

From caring, comes courage —Lao Tse

The Bunny Story

O*NCE* upon a time there were three little bunnies—a brown bunny, a black bunny and a white bunny. A long time ago they had been hurt and frightened, so all three bunnies went into hiding. The bunnies remained buried for a very long time while layers upon layers covered them. They had gone into hiding looking for safety, but after a certain length of time buried under the many layers covering them, they didn't know how to get out. Somehow they were able to survive and they loved and cared for each other deep within the ground. But they began to wish they could go outside again.

One day they heard a noise above them. The noise sounded like digging. It was a little scary because they were not used to hearing the noise. They listened carefully. Then, talking among themselves, the three little bunnies decided to be brave because they hoped that they really could get out. What they didn't know was that on the ground above them there was a friendly puppy who was digging off the layers. Now this puppy could smell the bunnies although at first he wasn't quite sure what they were. But he was a puppy who liked bunnies and would never, ever hurt them. So the layers began to come off one by one.

Under the ground, the bunnies began to see a dim light above them. They began to be excited and yet scared at the same time. It had been such a long time that they had been underground that they wondered what to expect. They all took a deep breath and decided to be brave no matter what, those three soft beautiful little bunnies.

The puppy, panting, would take a break to run around the trees, play and prance, and examine the flowers and plants as puppies do. But he always came back to continue digging through those layers. His sense of smell told him he was right, there were bunnies down there. His tail wagged faster and he dug furiously. He was excited and wanted to see some new friends. Pretty soon he broke through the earth and he stopped and sat, looking intently at the hole. The bunnies looked up and saw his eye looking down. Again they were a little frightened.

They called out, "Who are you?"

The puppy wagged his tail and said, "I wanted to help you. I want to be your friend."

The bunnies said, "You look awfully big and scary."

The puppy replied, "Yes, I guess I do look pretty big and scary, but I won't hurt you. Can you trust me?"

The three bunnies discussed this and decided they wanted to try to trust the puppy, but they agreed to be watchful. So they scooted to one side of the hole so the puppy could begin digging again. More layers came off. Soon the bunnies could see the light and it hurt their eyes because it had been so long since they had seen sunshine—but again they felt excited.

The hole got big enough for them to climb out. The puppy backed away, sat down, and watched. The bunnies stayed in the hole and looked out cautiously. It seemed a little scary to move out of their safe hole. They were unsure as to what to do. So, they decided that one of them would take a chance and come out. The soft black bunny stuck his nose—and then his whole head—out of the hole and looked around blinking. Sure enough, there was that puppy sitting there wagging his tail.

The little bunny said, "I have been in there so long, I don't know how to be. I don't know what to do."

The puppy nodded. Then he cocked his head, thought a minute, and said, "I have an idea. Why don't we push the leaves around the hole so that nobody else can see it. You can hop back and forth in here any time you get scared, yet you won't be buried among the layers.

The black bunny thought that was a good idea. He stuck his head back down in the hole and he said, "Come on out. It seems okay."

The beautiful little brown bunny stuck his head up, wiggled his nose and hopped out, shivering a bit.

The puppy came over and licked the brown bunny and said, "You will be okay. I will help you."

They said to the white bunny, "Come out. It's okay now."

So the white bunny climbed bravely out of the hole. The three bunnies sat looking around.

"It seems like a whole new world," said the white bunny.

The puppy nodded, understanding. "Yes, I suppose it would. I'm glad you're out."

The brown bunny said, "It looks like we're going to have to learn lots of new things." And they all nodded in agreement.

"Well," said the puppy, "let me show you some things. Follow me." He took them to a nearby garden with fresh plants growing. The top of the ground smelled so good! The bunnies happily munched some plants for a while. They noticed how warm and nice the ground was. They had forgotten how cold it was underneath the ground, but here it was warm and comfortable.

The puppy, watching them, noticed the white bunny was limping. "It looks like your leg is hurt."

The bunny nodded and said, "Yes, it got hurt a long time ago when we had to go underground. It never did heal right."

The puppy said, "I think I can help you."

He led them to where the water was and said, "Get in and rinse it off first." So the white bunny slowly hopped into the water, allowing the water to flow over the hurt, and then came out.

The puppy said, "Now hold still a minute. This may hurt a little bit but I need to lick the hurt because it will help it." Animals do that, you know.

Now the bunny was a little frightened that the puppy got so close but he reminded himself to be brave and trust the puppy. So he let the puppy lick his sore leg. He was surprised at the touch of the puppy's tongue. It felt good even though his leg was sore. Then the puppy scampered away again and brought back a special leaf which he put in the water to soften. With the help of the other bunnies, who had been watching closely, he wrapped the leaf around the brave white bunny's leg. The puppy said, "This is an old remedy that my grandmother told me about and it heals many things, so we'll try it on your leg."

He was a very smart puppy. The bunny was most grateful because it did start to feel better.

"Now you know," the puppy said, "when it starts feeling better, you will have to exercise it. You are going to have to learn new ways to use it." The bunny nodded bravely and said, "Yes, I know and I will work hard."

Then the puppy and the bunnies together found a new place for them to stay that was very safe. It was close to the garden, close to the warm earth, and in the warm sun. It was near their old hole too, in case they needed it.

The puppy said, "I will stay around here and help you and make sure there is no danger to you. I will show you which creatures and things to trust, and which ones to stay away from.

The bunnies snuggled up next to the puppy and they all loved each other very much. The puppy was very happy to have three new friends.

The Bunny Story is for everyone. It addresses the basic issues of fear and anxiety, which are common to all. The story encourages creating a safe place within yourself and promotes feelings of safety, nurturing, trust, and caring for others. The Bunny Story also encourages making choices and taking risks, exploring new things, working together, persistence in healing, growth, and courage.

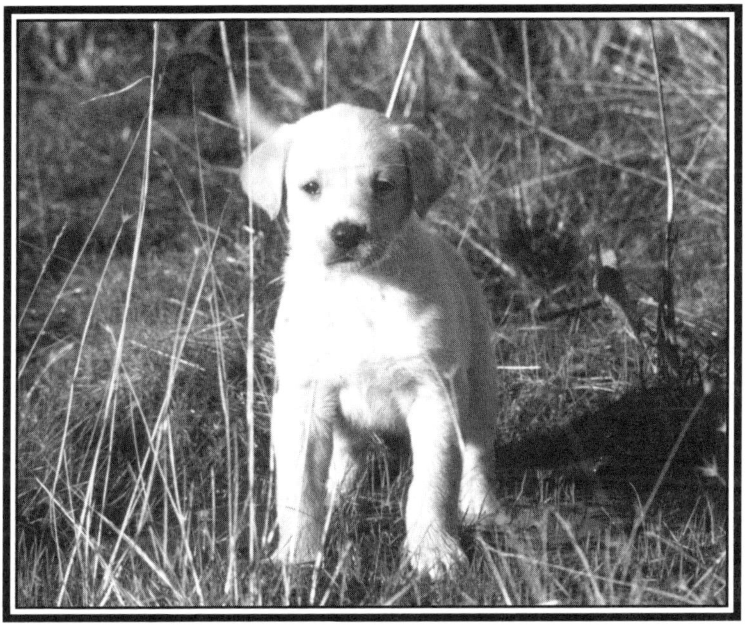

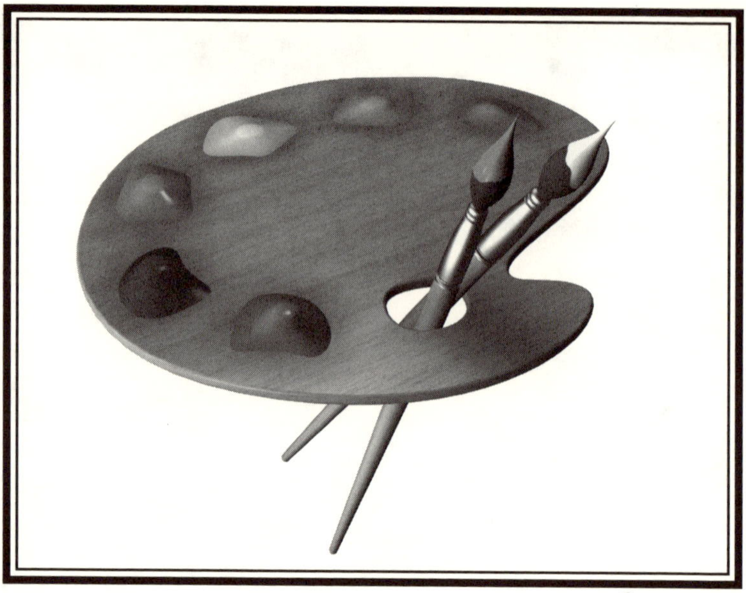

© Olga Rut'ko

Nothing will ever be attempted, if all possible objections must be first overcome.

The Young Painter

*O*NCE upon a time there was a girl, who had long, flowing hair. One day she decided to go on a journey. She began the journey by looking for, and finding the person who was in charge, for she needed permission to go on this journey. She found the old wise one who took both of her hands and gave her a blessing. "Go, my young maiden, and follow your heart. And remember to follow the tracks."

Now she was unsure, as she left what the wise one meant by that. She thought of the train tracks, and she thought of the car tracks, and she thought of the tracks that the animals made. She was puzzled about what kind of tracks she was to follow. She started off on her journey anyway and soon realized she was following a different kind of track. As she went on, taking steps to go on her journey, she saw an art center in the distance.

"How curious," she thought. "I wonder what this is all about."

When she reached the art center, she went inside. She found it was a place where there was much going on. It was not a museum. This was an active place where people were creating different things. All kinds of pictures were being painted. She wandered around, watching and occasionally picking up a brush herself. As she watched and learned, she realized how much she could do in painting a picture. She could select or rearrange different colors and make the picture look entirely different. She could paint objects bigger or smaller and that, too, would change things. She found it was possible that a different kind of background in a picture would change the feel of the picture. So she had great joy experimenting, trying new techniques.

She found it was possible to make dark things light, and to make dragons appear funny. There was so much she discovered that she could do with a paintbrush and some of the other tools. She also watched how each of the others painted their pictures. Some of the pictures were very similar and some were very different. Some of the pictures evoked emotions to make you feel many things, and some were simply interesting and curious. The young painter learned more than she ever thought she would learn. She was so happy that she had received permission to go on this journey. This was such an interesting place. Some people would tie things together that usually weren't tied together. For example, one person had painted a picture where an elephant was tied to a bunny rabbit. Now that was rather funny. But it was wonderful to notice that you can untie those things that shouldn't be tied together, with a simple stroke of the brush.

In another part of the art center, people were experimenting with different frames. Some people used brand new frames of different kinds of wood. There were many different shapes of frames. Some were simple, some were ornate. Some people liked to use old frames and refinish them. As she was watching one person, she noticed how easily this person was scraping the old gilt off the picture frame, part of the process of making it new. Underneath all the gold gilt was beautiful wood. The girl realized how many different frames there could be that would fit the picture that was being painted. She was having a marvelous time. This was a wonderful art center where you could choose to be in whatever room you wanted, and you could choose to paint in whatever colors you wanted for as long as you wanted

There were rooms for ceramics, and other kinds of materials. She had fun working with the clay. Everyone was going to the part of the art center that they wanted to. Some people would stay a very long time in one place. Other people would move about very quickly. It was nice to know that they had a choice.

It was very light in the center so that the magnificence of all the colors could be seen very clearly. There was always someone to ask for help if you wanted. There were all kinds of paper and each had a different feel. Some were very smooth and some were rough. The young painter had a marvelous time experimenting with it all. There were not only paints, there were many, many other kinds of implements, some of which she had never seen before. She was eager to try these new things. She felt very grateful that she was allowed to come here because this was a very special place, and everyone had come here with permission. She also found it was very easy to keep track of all her things, for there seemed to be a new system of doing that, which made it very easy.

So the girl decided to stay there for quite a while, for she loved the colors that she had never seen before. She loved that she could paint everything that she wanted. She would paint horses, or flowers, or cars or angels or nothing. The young maiden knew that she could continue her journey any time she wanted and could come back here. Or she could stay here as long as she wanted. While she was here, she painted a beautiful picture that she was going to give to the wise one who gave her permission to be here.

Leaving the girl to see with new eyes, to hear with new ears and to understand with a new heart, we see that whatever she did, she added to her paintings a special ingredient of love, which caused a glow in all of those who saw her work.

The Young Painter is about giving ourselves permission to explore our creativity. It helps us see options, make connections, and make choices and decisions. The Young Painter assists us in becoming comfortable with change and accepting joy in trying new things. This story helps us release unnecessary guilt and promotes helping others and listening to inner guidance.

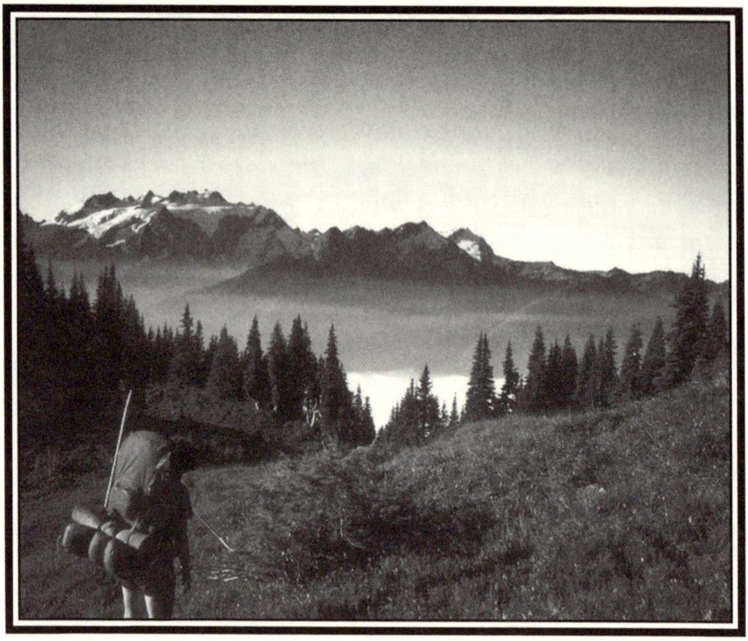

The real act of discovery is not in finding new lands, but in seeing with new eyes.

—Marcel Proust

THE BOY'S JOURNEY

ONCE upon a time there was a young boy who went on an adventure. He walked to a place where he had never been before. It was a strange land with many new and different sights. As he walked, he came upon an unusual elephant, green with yellow stripes. This elephant was stuck in the mud. This was a strange land, indeed. As the boy stood and watched, the elephant, as large as it was, was able to get out, and turned and looked at the boy. The boy understood how that was done and how the elephant was able to move on. The elephant learned also.

The boy continued on his way. He remembered that he had a camera with him. He took it out, looked into the viewfinder and noticed that something wasn't quite right. He couldn't see very well. He realized that someone had put a lens on the camera. Actually it was a zoom lens. He started to experiment with it. The boy realized that he could make those blurry images come into focus. Not only that, he could change the focus. Sometimes he could focus on something that was quite close, and at other times he could focus on something that was farther away. Since there were other lenses for this camera, he learned that he could focus on the smallest details if he wanted, or he could attach the wide angle lens. As he experimented with the camera, he got very good at knowing which lens to use, and when. He became very skilled in knowing how to operate the focus of each lens. He also knew which direction to turn and learned to change his focus quickly. Sometimes he would focus in one direction, then turn and focus in another direction. He had many choices.

Now, because the boy wanted to carry the camera with him at all times, he decided there were things in his backpack that he needed to remove. So, putting his backpack on the ground, he took everything out of it. The backpack held a lot. Some things were outdated. Some were no longer useful. He decided which things he wanted to keep and he was able to choose to leave behind the things he no longer needed. When he was done, there was plenty of room for the camera and new objects he might want. Putting the backpack back on, he stood up and was surprised to see that there were many directions that he could go.

He walked along making his choices, and he came upon a brilliant blue pond. Looking into the pond, he saw many bubbles coming to the surface. This was a beautiful pond. The water was very clear. It was very deep and he could see very far down. As he looked deep, he could see the bubbles being released and could watch them as they journeyed up to the surface. It was as if the bubbles carried something that he could not quite see. Some of the bubbles had different shapes than others. The boy had fun watching the bubbles come up to the surface and pop, releasing what was being carried there. In fact, it made him laugh.

When he decided to move on in this new and different place, he turned to the right and was surprised to find that there were several doors in a row. Skipping along, he ran and opened all of them. Behind the doors he found piles of rocks. He stopped and played with them as he did when he was little and played with blocks. He moved some of them one way and moved some of them another way, creating new patterns, and removing some from his way. Sometimes he walked around them and sometimes he would climb up and over. Then he might pick up some rocks and throw them far away. He had a good time creating new patterns.

Continuing his adventure, near the trees he found a spider web. It was quite intricate and he stood and looked at it. He noticed how easily the spider moved from place to place in the web. Other insects would get caught in the web. But the spider could run from place to place with ease. The boy wondered why the spider didn't get stuck. As he watched the spider, he saw that the spider knew exactly where she was going and what she was doing. She had a purpose after all.

As the boy continued his search, he found many interesting things. In some places he paused only a moment. In other places he stayed for a long time. He knew when it was time to move on. The boy felt connected to the trees, the rocks, the animals. It was as if he could feel how they felt. It was as if he could feel each and every thing that he looked at and touched. Even when he looked at the eagle flying high above, he could feel how it would be to be an eagle. When he looked at the smallest little bug crawling on the ground, he could feel how it would be to be that bug.

The boy had a marvelous time exploring. Once he came upon a little bunny that had been caught in a trap. He was happy to be able to let that bunny go free. This was a very special boy. He cared about the world and cared about this unusual land and the creatures here.

As he journeyed, he had fun using his imagination and found new interesting ways to do things that some people would find boring. He easily made friends with all the people and all the creatures that he met. It was as if he had an understanding far beyond what others did, and had knowledge from other places and times. And just like the bubbles, that knowledge would bubble up when he needed it. It was wonderful that this boy was so very happy.

The Boy's Journey helps us see life as an adventure, becoming open to new things thereby increasing our options. It assists in releasing the past, getting unstuck and finding ways around obstacles. This story helps us get out of ruts by shifting our focus and making different choices. It increases flexibility and connection to life. We can learn to put ourselves in others' places, increasing understanding as we listen to our inner voice. We can enjoy life and enjoy doing for others.

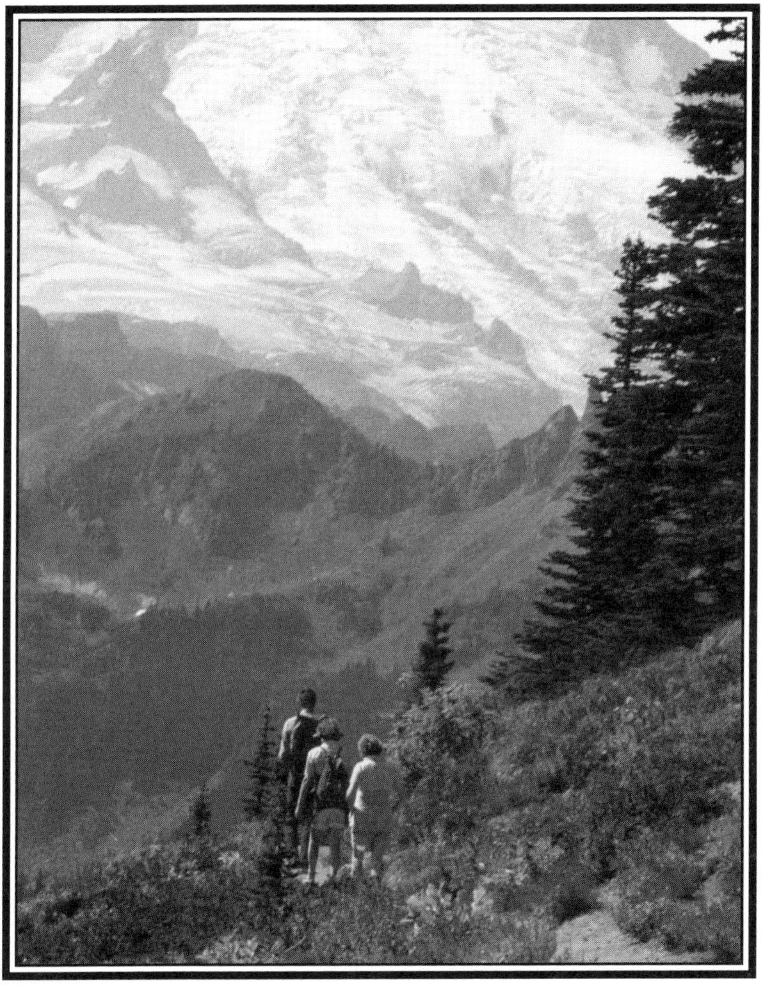

We cannot change anything unless we accept it.

—Carl Jung

The Critter

*O**NCE*** upon a time there was a furry little rabbit. The rabbit lived outside in a very large meadow with other rabbits who were his friends. He and his friends spent the days munching the tasty grass. The rabbit liked to sniff everything he saw, wiggling his nose as he took in the smells. Sometimes he would stretch out in the warm sun and take a nap. When he woke up, he played with his friends, hopping and racing across the field or playing hide and seek in the tall grasses and clover. He was a happy rabbit

One day, this furry little rabbit woke up and found something very different—a Critter on his back. The Critter was just sitting there.

"Well I don't like this at all," the rabbit said. "Hey, would you please get off my back?"

The Critter just sat there. So the rabbit got up and jumped up and down and tried to shake the Critter off. It didn't work. Then the rabbit hopped side to side and wiggled around. The Critter stayed on the rabbit's back.

"Get off my back!" shouted the rabbit. He was getting frustrated and angry, but it did no good.

"What are you doing? Why are you here?" the rabbit asked.

The Critter replied, "I want to be your friend." That surprised the rabbit because he thought the Critter was there to hurt him. "I can't be your friend," said the rabbit. "You are on my back and you aren't supposed to be there. It feels strange."

"But I like it here. Your back is furry and soft and warm, and it feels very good to me. I'm very comfortable here. I need a friend," said the Critter.

"But I don't want you on my back," said the rabbit.

"Yes, I know." said the Critter. "You will get used to me. I know we can be friends. I won't hurt you."

The rabbit ran around again, wiggling and hopping up and down trying to get the Critter to fall off his back. The rabbit bounded around and tried to scrape the Critter off by rubbing against a tree.

"But I need to be here for a while," the Critter said.

"Well, why?"

"Well," said the Critter, "I need to rest here for a while and besides, I like you."

"Humpf!" said the rabbit, "but you bother me." It was interesting to him that his friends didn't seem to mind at all. In fact they nodded and said *hi* to the Critter.

"I still don't want you up there", said the rabbit.

"But I can help you," said the Critter.

"What do you mean?" asked the rabbit.

"Well," said the Critter, "I'm higher up here so I can see where the good grass is and I can show you how to get there. Not only that, I can tell you if I see something that might be scary to you, like a dog or cat. Could I stay here for at least a little while?"

The rabbit thought about it. Although the Critter was annoying, the rabbit was beginning to like him.

"I'll give you a chance," said the rabbit because he was beginning to soften. "It's not real comfortable, but let's see how it goes for the next few days."

After a few days, the rabbit and the Critter became close friends and they did help each other. The rabbit liked having the Critter on his back. It made him feel safer and he had a new friend. Finally, he said to the Critter, "You know what? You can stay here as long as you need to."

"I appreciate that," the Critter said.

And they both knew that there might be a time when the Critter would leave. Until then the rabbit and the Critter enjoyed each other. The Critter showed the rabbit new places to go and suggested new adventures, and they were very happy.

The Critter is for accepting something necessary, for example a knee joint, a cast, a wheelchair, having to care for someone in your home or any other situation that you would rather not have. This story helps us give something a chance.

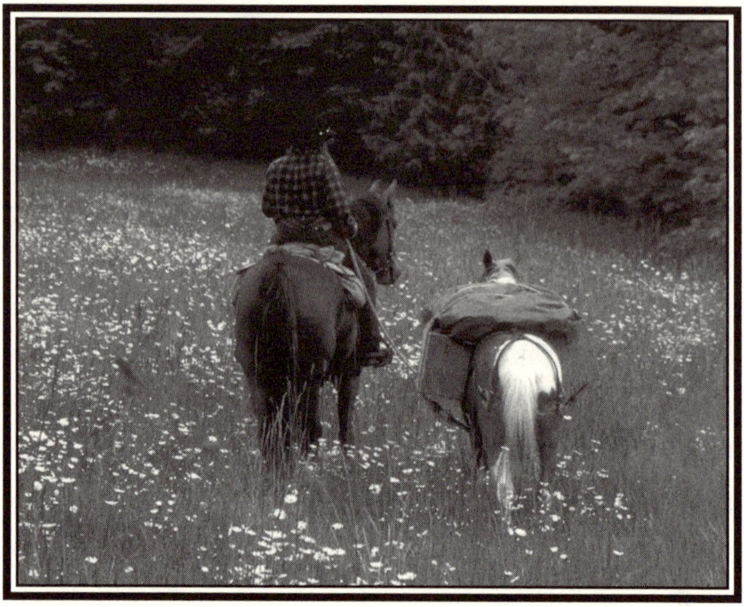

We can easily forgive a child who is afraid of the dark; the real tragedy of life is when men are afraid of the light.

—Plato

The Gentle Outlaw

ALL of the animals began to gather. They came to the central gathering place in the forest, for they knew that something important was about to occur. But they didn't know what it was. Even the ones who had never been to that special place before, were able to follow their instincts and find their way, even the skunks—and the lizards, as well as the coyotes—and the deer, and the wolves. For they knew this was a time to set aside their differences for what was about to take place.

One by one, or in twos and threes, over a period of time they all made their way to that very special clearing. Some of them had to come from far distances, and some of them had to travel over land and sea. But eventually they all arrived. Now of course, not all the animals could be there, but there was a spokesperson for each of the groups. They sat around looking at the campfire, night after night while they waited. Curiously, they weren't quite sure what they were waiting for. They knew only that it was important that they be there. While they waited, there was a violent rumbling of the ground beneath them. The volcano in the distance began to erupt—and floods began to appear. But still they stayed, waiting, for they knew it was important.

Suddenly, almost when they least expected it, *She* appeared. Now they had heard about her through legend, but not one of them ever expected to really be in her presence.

She said, "I have called you together here because I need to tell you all a story."

The animals listened expectantly, for they now knew that was why they had come.

"In a far away land, once upon a time, something terrible happened. The details aren't important," She said to the animals.

"What you need to know is there was much pain and much wounding, especially of the child. He became hysterical, this little child. Terrified, absolutely terrified. Screaming and crying and totally out of control. One day, an Outlaw happened upon this child.

"Now this Outlaw, well, he was a law unto himself. But something stirred within him as he looked at that child shaking, hysterical. He reached down from the horse upon which he was riding and swept the child up onto the horse, in the saddle in front of him. And he rode away with him.

"Now because the Outlaw was not all bad, really a gentle Outlaw, he took care of the child. In fact, he sort of liked the Kid. He settled the Kid down a bit, calmed his fears and got the Kid interested in the horse. And my, the child did like the horse!! Now the Outlaw did not ask many questions, just enough to know that he had really saved the child.

"So time passed. Although the Outlaw had rescued the Kid, some things that the Kid learned from the Outlaw weren't the most positive in the world to know. For the Outlaw was one who took over, did what he wanted. When the Outlaw was a child, he had not been guided well. So the Outlaw delighted in making his own rules, and looked with disdain upon the rules of the others in the land.

"One day, while riding with the Kid, the Outlaw got into trouble. And he became very, very angry. The Kid watched in amazement, for the Outlaw was acting just like he had when the Outlaw found him. The Outlaw began kicking and screaming and having a tantrum. The Outlaw was angry and terrified and hysterical. The Kid did not know what to do. For as long as they had been together, you see, the Outlaw was used to doing whatever he pleased and he could be very impulsive. Although the Outlaw really wasn't out to harm anybody, he certainly was not sensitive to others who were around him.

"The Kid liked this Outlaw because he had been very good to him at a time when he really needed it. He was afraid that his Outlaw friend would be killed. So he ran and ran and ran through the forest searching for—he didn't know what, but he knew he had to find someone who could help. On the way, he got tired and battered and bruised, but he kept running and running. He knew somewhere—somewhere out there was someone who could help.

"Finally he stumbled into a great large hole. He tumbled down and down this hole, until he landed at the bottom with a big thud. Picking himself up and brushing himself off, he looked around with amazement, for it was a beautiful place. Maybe, he thought, maybe there is someone here who can help me. He called out for help. Sure enough, the King of this place answered.

"'What can I do for you, little fellow?' the King asked.

"By now, of course, the little Kid had the attention of the Queen and the others too. So he told them the story about his Outlaw friend. The King nodded wisely.

"'Show me where he is,' the king said to the Kid. And putting on his disguise, he followed the Kid back to where the Outlaw was. The Outlaw was in terrible shape by this time and the Kid was very frightened of his friend. But the king knew what to do. He said to the Kid, 'This cannot go on!'

"Stepping in and taking charge, the King gently bound up the Outlaw and took him back to the King's place. It was a very, very different place. The Queen, by this time, had made preparations for the Kid who was scared. The Kid hoped that he had done the right thing but he was really frightened. The Outlaw was his friend, and the Kid needed to help him. The Queen picked up the little Kid and rocked him. (He had never been rocked before.) She gave him milk and cookies and sang some very special songs that made him feel better all over.

"Meanwhile, the Outlaw had been put in a room where he couldn't hurt himself or anyone. He too, was given something to eat. It was left by the door so that he could take it when he wanted. The food was a very special mixture. At first, of course, the Outlaw was outraged and slammed against the walls and shouted, 'No one can order me around. I make my own rules.' But he was safely kept in the room. After a while he began to get tired. The moon shone into his room, spreading its light on the bowl of food that had been left.

"The Outlaw went over to the bowl, looked at it, and decided to eat it. Something very magical began to happen because this was a very special mixture prepared for the Outlaw on instructions from the King. The Outlaw began to calm down.

"The next day the King went to the room himself. He asked the Outlaw, 'Are you a little more calm now?'"

"The Outlaw, still wary, said, 'What do you want?'"

"'I want to talk to you about the Kid,' said the King.

"At the mention of the Kid, the Outlaw's eyes brightened, for as I said before, he did like the Kid. 'What about him?' he growled.

"'It's time that this young fellow be sent to school,' said the King.

"With that, the Outlaw glared at the King.

"'But this is a very different kind of school,' said the King. 'In fact, it is a school that you, too, may attend. I think you might like it.'

Since the King was not pushing this onto the Outlaw, the Outlaw decided to see what this was all about. 'Maybe I'll check it out,' he said warily.

"'You may. Come with me,' said the King. 'However, I need to tell you that if you begin to get out of control, you will be immediately put back into this room.'

"The Outlaw took a deep breath and said, 'I understand.' There was something about this King—there was just something about him that the Outlaw respected.

"Well, the Outlaw and the Kid did indeed go to this new school. It was unlike any that either one of them had ever imagined. Many, many things were learned by both. They both really enjoyed learning. The Outlaw, on his own, decided to stay and live within the rules of this new kingdom, for he learned to love the King and Queen very much. Of course he and the Kid became great friends."

She stopped speaking to the animals and looked at them all. Deep within their hearts, they understood. Giving them each a blessing to take back to the distant lands, and giving each one a gift, she left as quickly as she had come.

The animals, each in their own way, went back with this new knowledge—the little ones crawling on the ground, the colorful birds flying in the air, the large animals and even the creatures of the sea—they all knew.

The Gentle Outlaw helps us deal the with rebel part within all of us that can get us into trouble, the part of us that gets angry, scared and out of control. This story helps us to learn self control, patience, love and calmness. It helps in honoring differences and working with others. The Gentle Outlaw assists us in accessing and nurturing our intuition and wisdom.

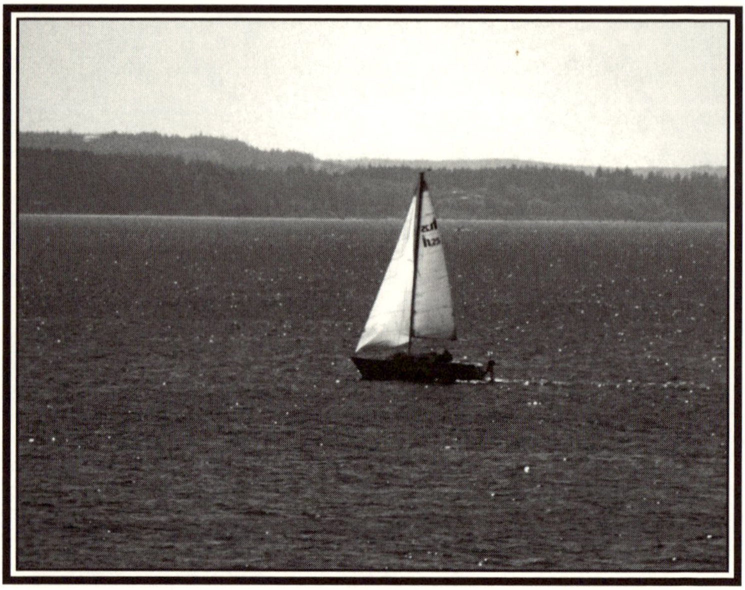

You cannot discover new oceans unless you have the courage to lose sight of the shore.

The Boat

*O**NCE*** upon a time there was a pretty little boat. This boat was tied up at the dock, gently and comfortably rocking with the waves, but the boat was feeling a little sad. It could not go anywhere because it was tied up. Occasionally the boat tugged at the line, hoping to get free, but didn't know how. It was tied up, going nowhere.

The child stood on the dock watching the boat, wishing she could ride on the boat. The little boat finally stopped struggling against that which held it, and noticed the child—finally focusing in a different direction.

"If you choose to untie me, we could go on a journey," said the boat.

The child thought about it and decided it would be an adventure. She found a way to untie the boat, for she was a smart child. As she stepped into the boat, it began to drift. Notice how it begins to drift, sometimes in one direction, sometimes in another.

"This feels so different than the feeling of being tied up," said the little boat. "I don't know quite what to do."

The child nodded but was not bothered.

"Why don't we just see what happens," she said, enjoying the drifting motion.

Now it may seem that the boat didn't know where it

was going, but as the boat quietly relaxed and allowed itself to drift, something new began to take place. The boat was now enjoying the drifting, feeling cradled by the deep ocean. It was very restful to feel the warmth of the sun, and hear the soft rush of the waves. That sound can be very peaceful and relaxing. Notice how the boat and the water almost seemed as one.

Deep within the mechanism of the boat there is a gyroscope, which keeps the boat balanced. The boat had forgotten about it, but soon, as the boat relaxed into the comfortable feel of the ocean, the boat began to feel the balance deep within itself, and knew there was guidance. The child noticed it too.

Now the child was enjoying her new adventure, exploring the boat, watching the waves. She jumped up and down excitedly when saw the dolphins. It seemed as if they came to put on a show just for her. She clapped her hands and threw them kisses because she loved them so much. The little boat was so happy to be able to share this with the delightful child.

Neither the boat nor the child noticed when the boat first turned toward a direction. The boat, in harmony with the water, chose a direction best suited for itself. The child found a compass that pointed the direction. It was there all the time. Even though the boat was adrift, at the same time it was on a course. But remember that it was necessary to untie the boat first. It was as if the water knew where the boat needed to go. The boat trusted the water to get it there.

The boat with the child journeyed to many different places and they learned many different things. Occasionally the boat stopped on different shores, and they experienced new adventures there, and then they went on, following the chosen direction.

The boat and the child went through many different kinds of weather. Sometimes the seas were very calm. Other times the skies turned gray and there might be a storm, with a lot of rain. It might seem uncomfortable but remember, the rain also cleaned the boat and made it look like new. Notice how stable the boat was as it rode through the storm. Sometimes the waves could seem very angry but all of this is a natural part of the seasons. The boat continued on the chosen direction, becoming gradually aware of its purpose, for indeed there were purposes.

Occasionally the boat needed to be put up on dry dock so that it could be overhauled. That meant sometimes the old paint needed to be scraped away, removing the varnish, removing the paint, removing the gilt or other unneeded decorations. The richness of the beautiful wood shone through as the new finish was put on. The child watched with interest. Occasionally planks were removed and replaced, so more major work could be done on the boat.

It is okay to be tied up in a harbor for a short time. It is possible to know when the time is right to set out to sea.

The boat received and carried many wondrous things to share along the journey. In fact, sometimes the cargo hatch was enlarged to hold more, therefore to give more. The child watched, participated, enjoyed. The boat was beautiful, strong and sturdy and very elegant. From time to time, new equipment was added to the boat when it was needed.

As the boat followed its natural course, the child was allowed to dive deep into the water to find the many treasures there. She loved exploring the beauty and majesty of the depths. The boat, by the way, also knew how to orient itself to the stars, and often navigated by them . . . following easily the natural direction. There were many ways of getting to the same place. It was very comforting and peaceful to be on the boat. It felt very safe. The child knew she could change directions and go home any time she wanted.

The child and the boat love to sail through the rainbows, lingering a while in each color. Each color has a different feel, the red, the orange, the yellow, the green, the blue, the violet. Yet though they feel different, they also feel the same. All the colors of the rainbow radiate peace, comfort, safety and strength.

The Boat addresses feeling stuck in life and also the feeling of drifting aimlessly and having no purpose. This story helps us to find our inner guidance, balance and stability. It assists in changing direction, opening to new adventures and experiences as well as getting rid of old useless patterns of thought, emotion (such as guilt), and behavior. The Boat helps us to weather the storms in life as we learn to develop trust in our intuition and find our path in life. This story is good for relaxation.

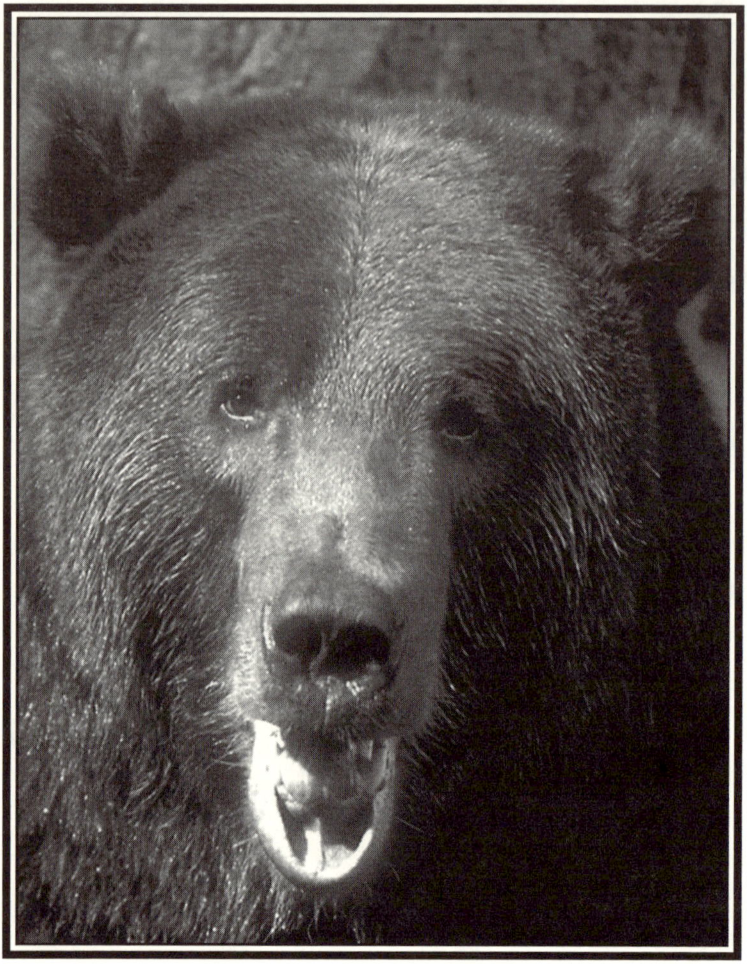

Courage is grace under pressure.

—Ernest Hemingway

The Bear

DOWN in a deep, dark forest, a little bear slept fitfully, sometimes sighing, sometimes whimpering in his sleep, for there was much going on in his little mind. He had been hurt when he was tiny, and he was very frightened. At last he awoke, gave a little bear stretch and his day began. He satisfied his hunger and his thirst and then continued exploring his world. As the sun warmed the air, the little bear, who had a loving and gentle heart, carefully stepped around the flowers in his path and he even stopped to watch a butterfly emerge. Presently, he came upon a cool pool of water. The little bear stepped closer to the water and stopped at the edge. Looking into the water, he was surprised to see a tear rolling down his face. He was lonely but that was okay. He brushed away the tear and he jumped into the cool water and splashed around, playing by himself. He did not notice the smiling unseen eyes around him. After a while, he crawled up onto a warm rock and took a nap in the sun. When he awoke, he noticed the sky had darkened as the clouds rolled in, and he decided to continue on his path.

Ahead of him, he heard a noise. The frightened little bear stiffened, his eyes hardened. His claws came out and a growl came out of his throat as he walked into the clearing. Some young cubs, took one look at him and ran away. So did the others. The little bear didn't understand. It happened all the time. "What's the matter with them?" he snarled. "Why do they always leave me out?" he muttered. Yes, it happened often. And he still didn't see the smiling eyes around him.

Much time passed, and with the passage of time, the bear hardened. The snarl and the scowl were there more often now. He even walked a little differently. He swaggered, and some would call it a little arrogance. Even so, he continued to step around the flowers and watch the butterflies.

One day on his journey, he crossed a bridge into another land, one where he had not been before. Something seemed different here, but he wasn't sure what it was. Shaking his head, he continued on, still not seeing the smiling eyes. By this time, the bear had endured much. His life had not been easy. Hearing a sound in the distance, he followed it. He came upon a waterfall and a deep, murky pool. He was glad, because he was thirsty. Looking into the pool, he almost couldn't recognize himself anymore. The face in the water surprised him with its frown and mean-looking eyes.

As he stood staring at the pool, staring at his reflection, suddenly there was another face in the water next to him.

He whirled around, claws out, snarling. To his surprise, there was a deer with soft eyes, and she didn't run.

"What do you want?" he growled. But there was no answer. Nervously, the bear pranced around and the deer simply followed. She motioned to the water with her head. For some reason, this frightened the bear and he jumped into the water and swam under the waterfall to the other side and got out. The doe followed, and motioned to the water again. Puzzled, the bear stared into the depths. He looked and looked and looked. This time he did not turn away. The murky water began to clear. The bear saw things he had never seen before. Tears washed clean paths down his soft face and fell into the clearing water. He sat down. The deer watched with her soft, smiling eyes. From time to time, the bear glanced up at the deer and she would nod encouragingly. He looked back into the depths and the tears continued, cleansing him. A light began to glow from the depths, began to glow stronger and stronger bathing everything in a wondrous mist of light. The bear felt and understood, as the water changed to a pure crystal clear allowing him to see many new and wondrous things. He sat for a long time, feeling the light. After a time, he looked up from the water, and the soft smiling eyes of the deer shone brightly. He now saw the smiling eyes of all the others. Then he smiled. Never again was the bear lonely. Although he continued to walk around the flowers and watch the butterflies, the snarl and growl were gone. He was greatly loved, and now he always saw the smiling eyes.

The Bear Story shows what happens when, experiencing fear, hurt, and anger, the bear isolates and becomes angry and hardened. This story addresses exploring the world, courage to look deep into yourself and cleansing old wounds by releasing the past. It promotes the courage to change, choosing to become increasingly aware of self and others. Gentleness increases as the heart opens, allowing the innate healing light to emerge. The world then looks different.

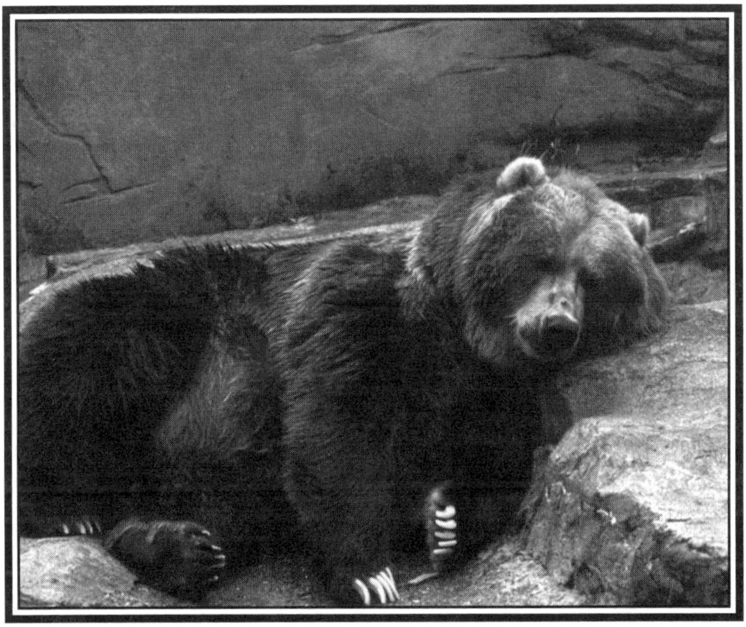

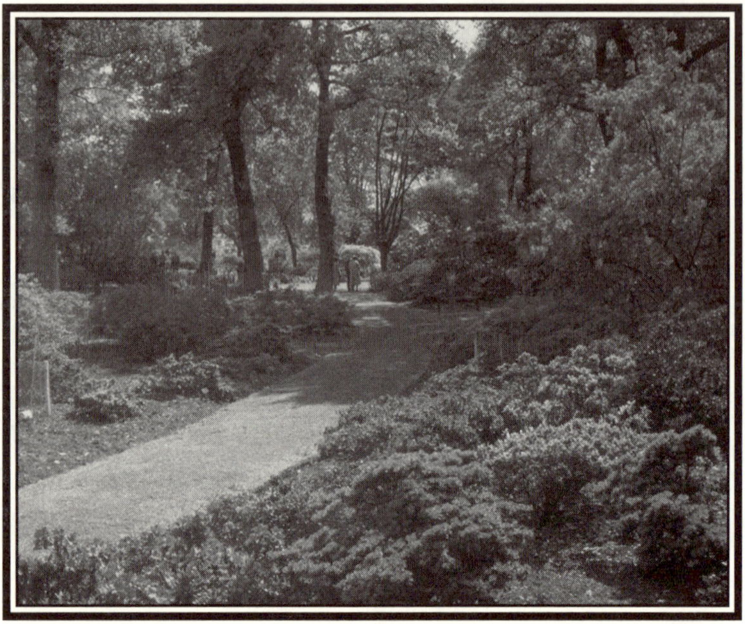

He who sows courtesy reaps friendship, and he who plants kindness gathers love.

THE CANS

I AM reminded of a story about a young girl. This young girl loved to be outdoors. She loved the feel of the sun on her face and the wind in her hair. She listened carefully to all the outside noises, the soothing chatter of the birds, the rustle of the bushes as a squirrel buried his food, the wind singing in the trees.

This young girl delighted in gardening. She enjoyed feeling the warm, rich dirt around her fingers and smelling the soil. She liked to talk to the flowers and the plants and to the earth itself. It was as if she could communicate with all things. When this young girl left the house, she had a habit of turning in one direction, climbing over rocks, sometimes getting scratched by the bushes.

One day she did something different. As she left to go to her garden, she turned in a different direction, and discovered a new plot of land. Taking her shovel, she began to dig there. What a surprise! She uncovered many cans. "How unusual," she thought. She rested and began to dig again and found more and more cans. Now these cans were of different colors and shapes. Some were blue cans, some were red cans, some had different patterns. Some cans seem to be old but there were many that were very new.

"What can I do with all these cans?" she thought. She

kept digging, fascinated by all of these cans. As she would pick them up, some of them felt very good in her hands. She looked at all the cans she had dug up and began to arrange them in patterns. Of course, there were some that she didn't want to use, but there were many that she did want to use, some because they felt good or she liked the shape or the colors or the patterns.

As she thought, she finally understood what she wanted to do with all these cans. "This will be my own very unusual garden," she said, and began to fill some of the cans with dirt. Then she began to plant seeds in these cans. Some of the cans she left here in this garden and some of the cans she took with her and decorated her other garden. It was interesting to note that there were new seeds that she had never planted before, and she put these in a few special cans.

Day after day, the young girl would come out and take care of her garden and would dig up new cans to use when she need them Her new garden began to bloom, and the colors of the flowers in these cans were magnificent. People for miles around would come to see her very unusual garden for it was quite spectacular. She was happy to share her joy and the beauty of her cans and flowers with everybody.

The Cans was developed for those people who see the glass as half empty, and think they 'can't' (can't do something, can't try something new, etc.). This story helps us to look under the surface of our lives and find the richness that is there. The Cans encourages us to appreciate nature and to be creative, responsible and sharing as we explore new directions.

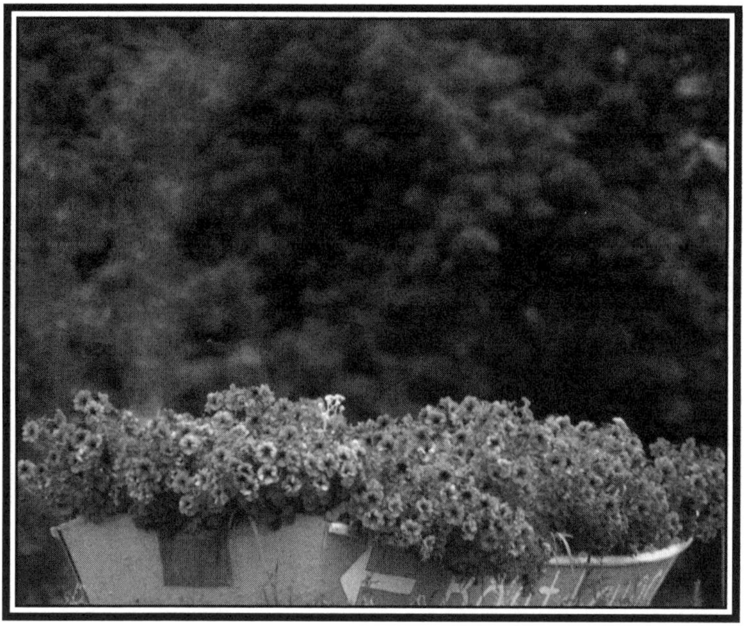

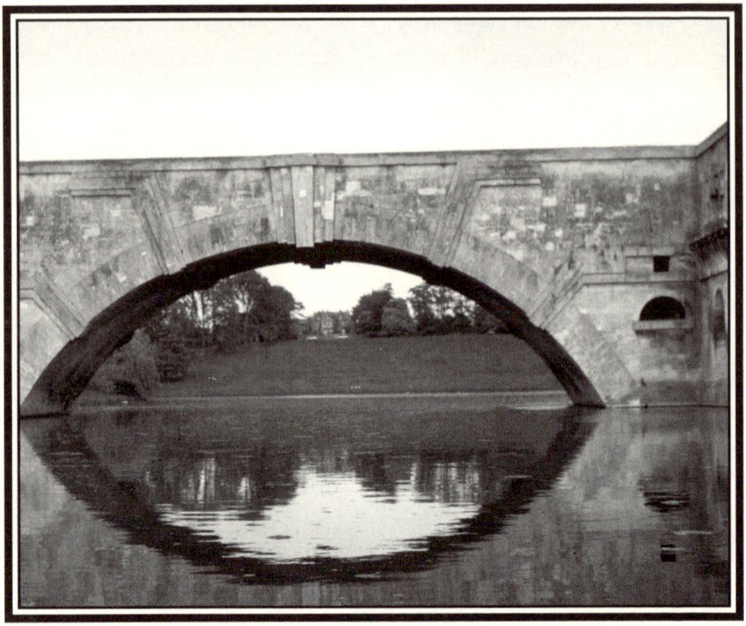

Don't be afraid to take a big step if one is indicated. You can't cross a chasm in two small steps.—David Lloyd George

The Magic Bridges

*O**NCE*** upon a time there was a small country, pure and peaceful. The people lived in simple loving harmony, caring about and helping each other, sharing and teaching. But one day a great calamity came upon this small country, the effects of which lasted a long, long time. Hideous monsters marched through the land. These terrible monsters came from both outside the country and from deep within. The monsters caused great confusion. They caused great pain to the land and the people, including the children. The people battled valiantly, striving to protect their land and people and the children.

The monsters were very clever in their destruction, causing things to be turned upside down. They caused great sadness and pain. Since the monster attacks continued for many eons, the people of the land no longer knew what was true and began to battle among themselves. The monsters left this country leaving great damage behind. The people no longer knew each other, and they continued fighting bitterly. The children also had been hurt and they too, were confused. Connections between the people were broken and bridges had been destroyed.

Deep within a way-off forest in this small country, something began to stir. For hidden deep within a cave, a girl-child had been born with great wisdom. This girl-child had been sent from afar and had knowledge from beyond this place. Even the animals knew there was something special about this child and protected her fiercely, working together in agreement to keep her hidden. In the cave with her, unseen by all except those who had special vision, were several large angels who ministered to the small child.

One day it was time for her to emerge from the cave, for she had grown stronger and bigger. Time for additional lessons had begun. One angel told her that she had a special mission: to bring peace and healing in the land, for the girl had been born with great love in her heart.

"How?" the child asked. The angel smiled and began training her in the secrets of the universe. By night, the angel appeared as a beautiful snowy owl and led the girl to secret wisdom places of the universe. Only the animals and fairies knew of the child and her training, keeping the secret and protecting her. The training continued for a long time.

Finally she was ready, matured by the timeless wisdom and disciplined training. Accompanied by the unseen angel she left the forest and went out into the land. She was greatly saddened by what she saw. Being wise, she traveled for many years until she knew all of the problems. She met and listened carefully to all of the warring people and saw all the devastation.

When the timing was right, she began using ageless wisdom she had so diligently learned. Gradually the warring people began to notice. The people watched with both awe and suspicion as she went about her work. She built many bridges across the land, the likes of which had never been seen before, for these bridges had colors and sounds of another time and place. At first the people ran away from the bridges in fear and anger. The young girl patiently continued her work, sowing her magic throughout the land, for she knew the bridges would be used when the time was right. For a long time, she was the only one who used the bridges. The people watched. In fact, they became so curious that they began to forget about fighting. The children began to come out of hiding to watch, even though some had been terribly hurt and badly frightened.

The special nature of the girl and her wisdom began to affect the people, and she knew that healing had begun. One day, one of the little boys had just had it! He had been one of the very angry ones, but his curiosity about the bridges became too much to resist. He came out of his hiding place defying the others and ran to the nearest bridge. This took great courage on his part. As he reached the bridge the special colors and sounds reached to his depths and he became transformed in a way that had never been seen. He ran onto the bridge, stopped, tested it with his feet, then took off his shoes to feel the material. At last, he looked out and saw the land in a new way. The people also suddenly saw something different about the boy. With joy, he ran to the other side of the bridge where he met those whom he used to fight. Word of his courage spread throughout the land. Slowly at first, a few others began approaching the bridges, then more and more. Connections began to be made between the people. The fighting ceased as the magic and wisdom of the girl and her bridges began to work their miracles. Love and joy returned to the land and the people once again began to work in harmony, appreciating each others' uniqueness. The confusion left and once again the people knew what was true. Best of all, the children were healed. The girl, the unseen angel, and all the animals were content.

The Magic Bridges helps with the pain and chaos both without and within. It gives us hope as we access our inner wisdom and spirituality. The Magic Bridges teaches us to objectively look at problems before acting, trust in universal timing as we persist and develop listening skills, courage, patience, discipline and love. It helps point us to connecting with others, peace and harmony.

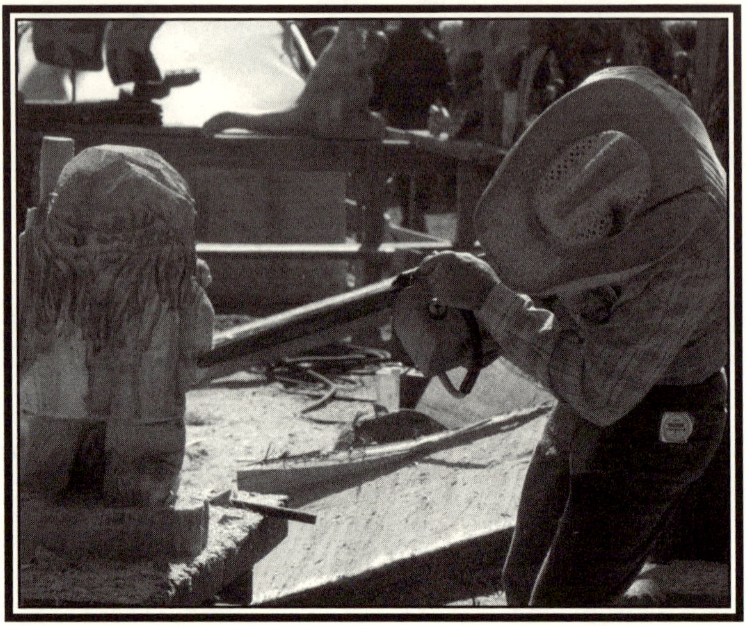

It is not because things are difficult that we do not dare, it is because we do not dare that things are difficult.

—Seneca

The Woodcarver

ONCE upon a time there was a village. This was a very interesting village, for it was filled with artists and craftsmen of all kinds. The people of the village made beautiful work and they loved what they did. It was the custom in this village for the children to learn crafts from the fathers or mothers and the teachings were handed down generation to generation.

In this village there was a woodcarver who made magnificent furniture, with unique joints and patterns. The patterns of this furniture were family patterns, which the woodcarver handed down to his son. The furniture was strong, very solid and some of the most admired for miles around. The son enjoyed learning how to make this furniture and the magnificent woodcarvings from his father. The son, too, made very solid and beautiful furniture from these family patterns.

While he was working, because he was so skilled, he would often daydream. When he would allow himself to daydream, he would see interesting new patterns in his mind, patterns never seen before. However, since he was to follow the family patterns in his work, he didn't feel that he could use these patterns that he was seeing in his mind.

The son became more and more unhappy and he didn't know why. He enjoyed his work and his family and did not know why he wasn't happy. He began not to be able to concentrate and wondered, "What is wrong with me?" Pretty soon he became very sick and couldn't work. Everyone around him was concerned because they loved and cared about him very much, plus he was such an excellent craftsman. No one knew what was wrong. His family was concerned, and even the little girl that loved to watch him make furniture wondered when he would get better.

One day they called upon the wise man of the village to come for a visit. The wise man came in, looked at this sick young man and sat next to him. The wise man put his hand on the young man's shoulder, for that gave him a lot of information. By now, the son was so sick he was not getting out of bed. The father stood in the doorway, looking very concerned. And the little girl was sitting on the floor at the foot of the bed. The mother was standing at the side of the room and you could tell she was praying for the health of her son. They all kept quiet while the wise man was there.

After a while, the wise man spoke, looking directly into the young man's eyes. He said, "Craftsmanship is very important, and you do lovely work, but sometimes patterns need to be broken. You will not be well until you also build the patterns of your dreams." With that, the wise man got up and left.

The son said to the father, "But I need to carry on the family patterns."

The father said, "My son, we want you to be well and happy. Think about what the old wise man said."

The son began to allow some of those dreams and patterns that he had once seen, to float through his head again. They were beautiful patterns of shapes and colors that had never been thought of before. As he simply allowed those thoughts to go through his mind, he began to feel better.

It wasn't long before he was well enough to be up out of bed for a little while. His family began to get smiles on their faces, for they loved him very much. And the little girl continued to hang around. He decided that he might try to build something following the pattern in his mind. He looked at the little girl and decided to start with a small chair for the her. Using the new pattern in his mind, he began to build this small chair. Because he was such a good craftsman, having practiced a lot, the chair was strong and sturdy...and very lovely with the new pattern that had never been seen before. The little girl was delighted, happy with her new chair. The father was very proud of his son.

Now the son builds dream furniture. Everyone wants his dream furniture. First he will dream and then he builds. It has an extra quality to what he builds because of the dreaming. It is the same excellent craftsmanship. Beautiful. The son still uses the family patterns and still hands them down. But now he has a choice of which family patterns he wants to build, and when. He is very happy as he builds his dream furniture, using the new patterns. Everyone in the village is delighted for they, too, benefit. The son is known far and wide.

The Woodcarver increases our creativity and learning. It helps us break old patterns and honor both the new and old. It encourages choice and responsibility. The Woodcarver encourages us to find the wise part of ourselves and to follow our own unique paths, appreciating the creativity, which can be found everywhere.

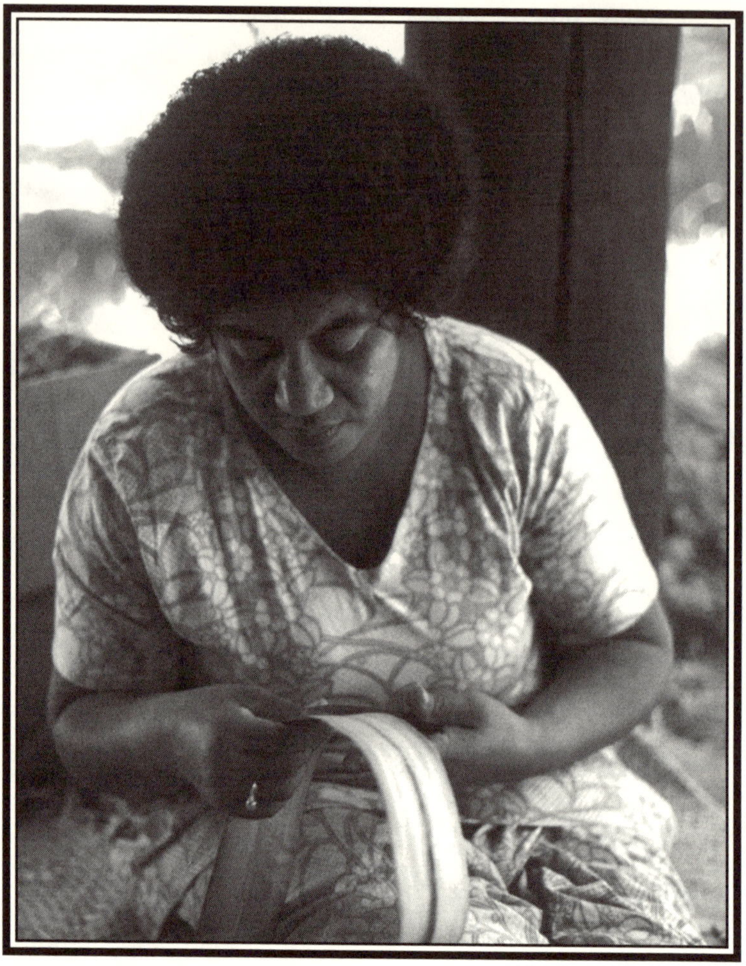

With time, all is made right.

The Mender

*I*T is beautiful to walk among the trees on a fall day and watch the leaves gently float to the ground because it feels and looks so restful. It is as if the trees know how to get ready for a time of rest. As the winds turn cool and the fall air changes, the trees naturally respond. The leaves change into glorious colors and when the time is right, one by one the tree, in agreement with the leaves, releases them. During winter, the trees rest. Notice how they have their own kind of beauty even when the snows come. All of the seasons are beautiful. In winter also, there are animals who hibernate, crawling into their special places. Other animals seem to become more alive in the winter. In the snow there are many, many different kinds of tracks. Sometimes you can follow one kind of track and other times you follow other kinds of tracks. There are always tracks you can follow. What fun it is to discover all the wondrous things that you did not know were there. For it is possible to find things in the winter that you had no idea about in the summer.

It is soothing to watch the mountain stream as it makes its way down the mountain. Notice how the water flows around the rocks and sometimes it flows over the rocks. If there is something very large in the way, the water knows how to find a different direction and is able to change its course, still continuing on its way.

It is fun to watch a small child at play with blocks. If these are large blocks, the child can build them very high. Notice how the child can move the blocks, making different patterns. Sometimes the child can place the blocks all around, so he is inside. But it is easy to push the blocks out of the way when the child wants to get out. How easily the blocks can be moved.

When you watch an eagle in the sky, it is indeed a beautiful sight. The eagle freely glides on the wind currents as if the eagle can rest on them. Such strength and power are in those wide wings. How freely the eagle glides across the sky and circles. It is so good to be free. The eagle can see very far in all directions—farther than we can. Yet the eagle can also focus and see something very small. What fun it is, and the eagle knows when to shift the focus.

Once upon a time in a village far, far away there was this lady with very special gifts. She could mend anything that anyone brought to her. From far and wide, people of the countryside brought her things to mend, for she had a reputation of being able to mend things so that they were stronger than before. Children would bring to her their toys to mend. Little girls and boys brought roller skates, trucks, bicycles, dolls and kites. She knew just what to use to fix these items. It was almost like magic, how the mender did her work, knowing exactly what kind of material needed to be used to fix the broken item. She could mend all these different toys so that they were even better than new. Adults also brought things for her to mend, for she had a marvelous talent and could fix anything. The men of the countryside would bring their broken machinery, and somehow she knew how to fix them so they were strong and sturdy. She also knew when the timing was right. For example, some of the materials she used to fix things needed to sit in the sun for a period of time. She knew exactly the time that was needed, and still she was able to fix things faster than anyone in the entire countryside. Everyone also came to her for advice because she could mend more than objects. They listened carefully to her advice because she knew instinctively how to suggest repairs. The people of the countryside gave freely to her for they were so grateful for her work. Although she never charged for the mending she did, somehow she always had more than she needed, and was well loved by everyone in the village.

It is amazing to know how much can be accomplished when we least expect it. All we need to do is to listen and tune in. Even when we don't, it is accomplished anyway. How quickly time can pass when we want it to.

The Mender is for repairing things, from ideas, attitudes, relationships, to problems with the physical body or emotions. The Mender helps us access the part of us that knows how to do it. The images at the beginning point out the value of natural timing, shifting perspectives, and resting.

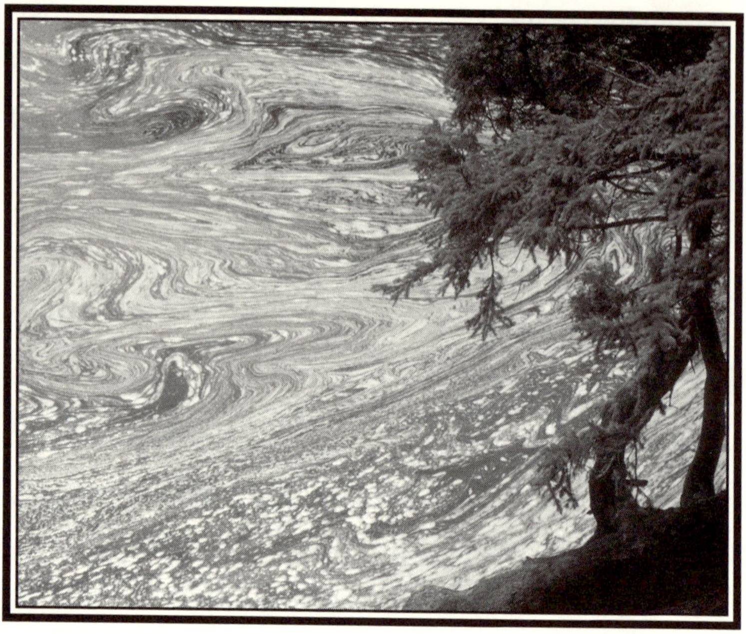

Life isn't a matter of milestones, but of moments.

—Rose Kennedy

The Tree's Life

THE tree had a wonderful view, standing high on a cliff overlooking the ocean and the beach. Even from this point, the tree could hear the sound of the ocean. That soothing sound. The tree loved the sparkle of the sun on the calm water, so peaceful. From his vantage point, the tree could watch all that was going on on the beach. Sometimes there was a lot going on, and other times it was quiet. Even in the midst of the activity, there was a certain peace. Sometimes a slight breeze ruffled the leaves of the tree. At other times, storms that would blow in with dark clouds, lightening and the loud voice of thunder. The tree liked it all. The tree was very sturdy. Notice how the roots grow deep into the earth. The tree liked the feel of the earth. The tree wiggled the roots around, growing them strong and deep as he took in nourishment from the rich soil. Notice how healthy the tree is as it takes up just the right nourishment for itself. The tree liked the feel of its roots going around the rocks in the dirt and saying hi to all its friends living in the earth, working together as a team. Sometimes the tree would tell those under the ground about the storms, for they did not know about them. The place where the roots grew was very quiet, no matter what happened above ground. The tree loved its roots and its branches that reached high in the sky. The tree loved its leaves, shimmering with the breeze, reaching toward the sun, feeling the warm sun on its leaves and branches. Because its roots were so strong, the tree felt as if it could reach forever.

Sometimes a lot of activity went on in the branches. Birds would arrive, build new nests, and have conversations. The tree thought some of the conversations were very funny. The tree loved watching its leaves move gently, and even move wildly when the storms came. The tree loved it all, all its experiences. It could see very far as it looked out over the beach and the ocean. Sometimes, the tree focused very near, watching a bug crawl up its bark, for it welcomed all.

The tree felt very calm inside and the feel of its strong core was a great comfort to the tree. The tree was wise for it knew that everything was in divine order. The tree was also patient, even with those pesky kids who came to climb it. Now normally he liked kids climbing through his branches but some of them became pesky, especially when they wanted to carve up his bark. But he accepted even that, being very accepting. If one of those kids got a little too rough, the tree would give a shake and the child would calm down. How beautiful it is, the tree thought, to be who you are.

One evening, the tree was reflecting on how natural his health and his growth came from that tiny seed. It was obvious that the seed knew exactly what to do. In fact the tree was in awe of the whole process. He was thinking, isn't it amazing how each type of seed knows exactly what to do. Each tree was different, unique, even if they were in the same family. He felt very close to all those other trees. In fact he felt very close to the rocks, the creatures underneath the ground, the birds. He even felt close to the kids. The dolphins that he could see, splashing in the ocean made him smile. The tree would nod to the magnificent whales in great respect for the messages that they carried.

The tree was very happy, serene, and content with his life. Not that he minded changes. He loved the seasons. In summer, everything was in full bloom, the leaves shimmering and sparkling as if waving to everyone. He loved the fall, when the leaves turned colors and changed. He loved each and every leaf, but he was not sad to see it go, for he knew the next season he would have new leaves. So as the leaves released and were carried on the wind, the tree happily wished them a wonderful journey, wherever they went. Sometimes the leaves would go slowly and sometimes the leaves would go fast, especially if there was a storm.

When the leaves were all gone, he peered up into the branches and thought how beautiful the empty branches were. I'm very gorgeous, he thought, but without any false pride. He just knew who he was. Being without leaves allowed him to see the branches and the whole structure of who he was more clearly. If the children would climb on his branches at that time, sometimes they would put decorations in the branches. It made him chuckle. Yes, he thought, I worked hard at accepting all that is.

He also marveled at how everything worked, for even if one of those bad beetles came, burrowing and eating part of him, he marveled at how quickly his whole being would take care of it in a right and proper manner. He swayed with comfort in the breeze, enjoying the storm clouds which were now upon him. He marveled at the beautiful light show of lightening and thunder, enjoying the cleansing rain and feeling the trickles that tickled as they found their way to the ground. The roots were delighted at all the new water. If things washed away a bit, the tree would give a shake to settle in and get comfortable again. Sometimes the storms were long, but they always seemed short to him. As the clouds moved away, he waved and thanked them. The sun came out to dry him, making things sparkling and new again. In winter, he liked the cold and the stark look of his branches. He liked it if there was snow on his branches. A new decoration he would say. The ocean that sometimes seemed calm and peaceful would at other times look rough and choppy. But the tree knew that the ocean had a core like his own and underneath it was strong and smooth. He liked the visiting boats that would come now and then. Sometimes he would see the people pointing up to him, for he was indeed magnificent. Some of the people came up to visit. Some of the people would call him *he* and some would call him *she* and it didn't matter to the tree, for the tree knew it was neither he nor she, but a tree. One day the tree experienced something new—an earthquake. *Well, isn't that interesting,* he thought. *That shakes things up good.* And isn't it interesting that after the shake up, the tree noticed things he hadn't noticed before, and was very pleased for that shake up. It reminded the tree that he was very strong and could survive anything. Calm and peaceful.

The Tree's Life is about self acceptance, appreciation, and self-esteem. This story helps us to be grateful for life and its many facets. It assists us in acknowledging our strength.

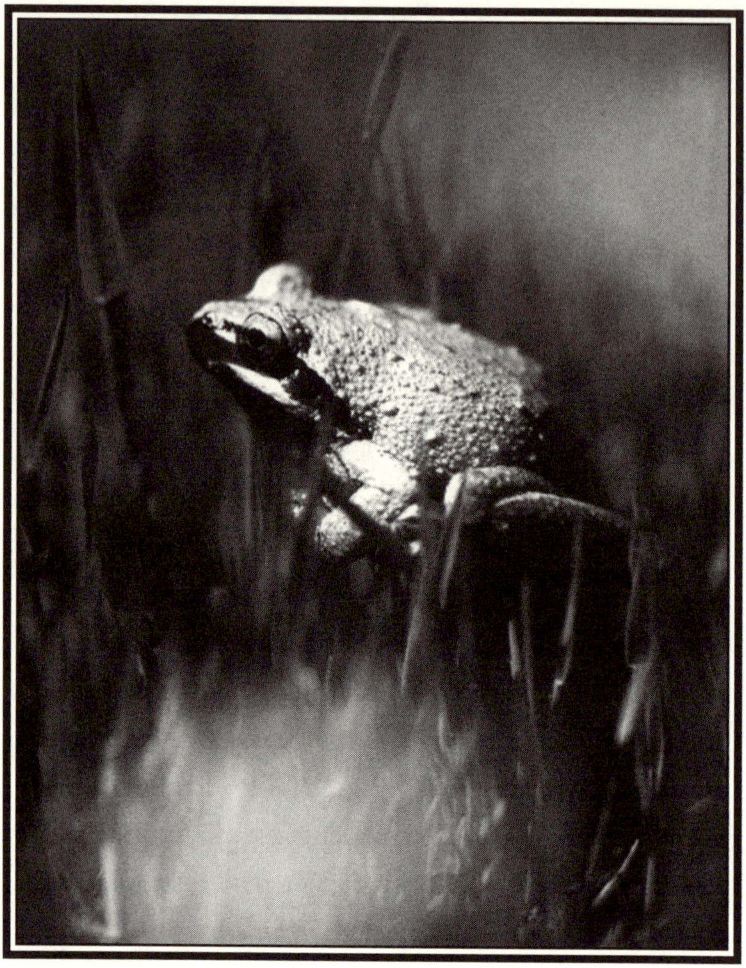

There are days when you don't have a song in your heart. Sing anyway.

—*Emory Austin*

The Frog Story

THIS is the story about a village of frogs. Once upon a time there was a group of frogs, some big, some little—a whole community. They had old frogs and they had very young tiny frogs. They were a loving community and liked each other a lot. They watched out for each other and took care of each other. These frogs all liked to croak. They loved the sound of their voices and each other's voices. They would croak by themselves when they were alone, and sometimes they would all get together and croak. Their croaking was like beautiful singing. All the voices were different. Even the little tiny frogs loved to croak with their little voices. The frogs would play and sing day and night.

One day something scary came through the woods. All the frogs were frightened and they scattered in different directions, hiding in many places. After a while, the scary thing left and all was quiet. But the frogs were lost from each other and they were all scared. Some of them could no longer make noise, but just lie in their hiding places, shivering. After a while, one of the bigger frogs began to croak. He wasn't sure that the big scary thing was gone, but he took a chance.

"I've got to find everyone," he thought. He croaked and he croaked, and then he stopped to listen. He didn't hear anything. He croaked and he croaked and it was very quiet. He ventured from his hiding place and hopped around a little bit. He began to croak again. Pretty soon, far away, he heard an answer. Excited, he hopped in the direction of the voice and croaked some more. By following the answering croak, he found one of his friends. They were so glad to see each other, for it felt as if they had been away from each other for a very long time.

"We must find everyone," they said to each other. Together they would croak and then listen. Croak, then listen. They would hear a voice and then find another frog. Some of the ones they found were the old ones. All of the frogs worked very hard and, one by one, they found their friends—the big ones and the little ones. They did not stop, all day and all night. More and more were found. Some of the little ones were still too scared to croak. Some of them had left a trail. The wise ones followed that trail. The scared ones were eventually found, and they were so happy. Finally, they stopped and counted. No, they still were not all found. There were still a few small ones missing.

"They must be very frightened," the frogs said to one another. They decided as a group, to search and search until every one of them had been found, no matter how long it took. They realized that it was important to have every one of them found. So they made a plan. They went in different directions in groups of three, croaking then stopping to listen carefully. It was very hard work. Suddenly, one of the older frogs said, "Stop, I thought I heard a noise." He made one croak and stopped, listening intently. Sure enough, he heard a tiny noise. It seemed to be coming from under a pile of leaves. The frogs hopped over, looking under leaves. They croaked, then stopped and heard the noise again. They began digging under the leaves, and way down under the leaves was the last tiny frog, scared and shaking. They were so glad to see him. They put him on the back of the biggest frog and told him he was safe now. The danger was over. Announcing with their loudest croaks that they had found him, they went back to the meeting place, all of them croaking loudly. Finally, the whole group was back together. They were so happy because it had been a very frightening experience. They all examined one another and told of their experiences. Some of them had been hurt but the older ones cared for them. During their conversation, the one of the teenage frogs told the group that while looking for the last frog, she had found a place that would make a great new home for all of them. It was very safe. "Would you like to see it?"

"Oh, yes," the wise ones said. The teenage frog led the way and the group followed her. It turned out that they were all very pleased. The new place was beautiful. There was a flowing stream where they splashed happily in the water. There were big lazy ferns and even a log to play on. There were places where they could play hide and seek. They examined this new place carefully and decided they would make this new place their home, for it was a place that was very safe from anything scary. Once again the frogs croaked loudly and happily in celebration. Even the tiny ones began to regain their voices, a little at first, but as they felt better, they croaked more enthusiastically. They had a marvelous celebration, singing and croaking, joyous that they were all back together again.

The Frog Story shows us the importance of finding our 'voice,' expressing who we are. The story assists in finding different parts of ourselves when we feel lost. The Frog Story demonstrates working with others for a common goal, the value of persistence and appreciating and respecting differences.

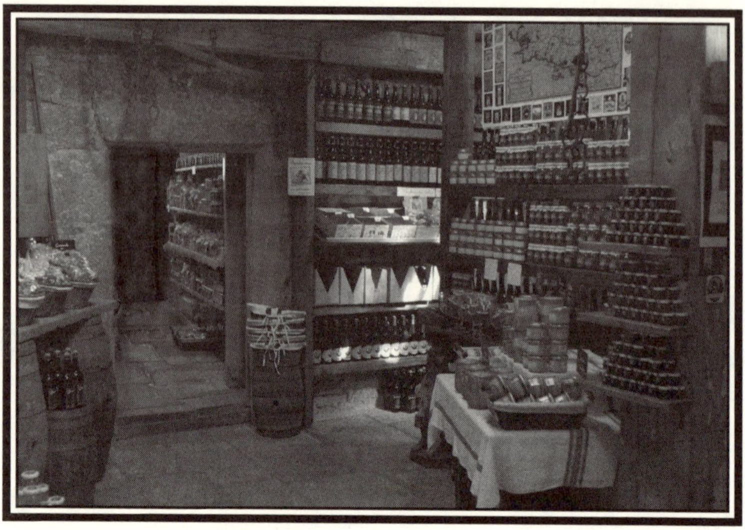

© *Marc Verdiesen*

Be the change that you want to see in the world.
—Mahatma Gandhi

The Alchemist

You take the key from your pocket. The key fits in the lock of the wooden gate that leads to your garden. Putting the key in the lock, you enter your garden. It is a beautiful garden with rich soil and flowers of many different colors. Colors of a variety of hues and brilliance and some colors that seem very different from those you normally see. In your large garden there are many varieties of plants and flowers in various stages of growth. Some are in full bloom showing their magnificent colors. Some are in an in-between stage. Some of the plants are very young and there is a section where the soil has been freshly turned, nourished and new seeds have been planted. This is a garden where you can come and rest. Looking around your garden, way at the other end, you see another gate with a large window in it. You make your way toward it, and there is a sense of excitement. As you move closer, you find yourself looking through your creative window. On the other side is a cute little white kitten. If you choose, you may open and go through the gate. As you go through the gate, you feel a strong easterly wind pick you up and gently carry you into your creative world. You may bring the kitten with you, or you may leave her where she is. She is a veteran of these creative trips and may prove to be a helpful guide.

The easterly wind deposits you on the ground and you find yourself in a large ancient laboratory. In front of you is an old man who seems not to notice you at first because he is very busy. It seems as if the little white kitten has been here before and she knows the old wise man. As you begin to adjust to where you are, you notice that he is surrounded by shelves and shelves of bottles, each one labeled neatly and precisely. He seems to be picking and choosing bottles from the shelves. You sense a certain wisdom radiating from this old man. He is what the ancients would call an alchemist. It is said that the alchemist knew the secrets of making gold, of combining ingredients that cannot be combined. As he continues to pick different elements, different substances, different ingredients, you may notice that you are familiar with some of these elements, like salt, silver, crystal powder, things that are found on earth. You look again, and you notice that he has bottles on his shelf containing every emotion, every feeling possible. He also has colors and essences of colors. You may be surprised at other elements that he has in his vast lab. Occasionally he will take a bottle, open it and sniff its contents as if that, too, were very important. Sometimes he mixes according to the aroma. Some ingredients in the bottles appear solid, but others contain what looks like a colored mist or fog As you approach the alchemist, he turns. In his eyes, you can feel his gentleness and his wisdom. He asks you what you want. You think for a few moments before you answer. He nods and he asks you to go to each of the shelves and pick those elements that you would like him to combine. If you happen not to have anything specific in mind, he will look at you very carefully, and he will choose for you from the shelves. He can make a potion, or a salve or some other form that you need. It's very interesting to watch him put all these things together. It is not long before the old wise man has combined what you need. With a loving look from his wise and kind eyes, he hands it to you and nods for you to use it. When you have finished, you may thank the alchemist for his talents and knowledge which you know have helped you in many ways. You allow yourself one last look into those loving eyes. As you turn to leave, you may notice a tremendous feeling of healing...physical, mental, emotional, and spiritual. Every cell in your body vibrates with youthful energy. You move back toward your creative window, and you notice a different attitude, a spring in your step, a feeling of joy, contentment and peace. Saying goodbye to the white kitten, you allow a gentle northerly wind to bring you back into your beautiful garden. You stop for moment to touch and feel the soil, put your feet in the ground, and touch the plants around you. You are feeling very connected and grounded in your world. After moving back through the garden and then through the gate you turn, and with your key, secure the gate, feeling very well connected to the ground, the garden, the kitten, the potions, the colors, the emotions, and the Alchemist.

The idea of The Alchemist is Transformation. In life we need to allow room for the unusual, the non-linear, the miracle. The Alchemist gets us in touch with that magical transcendent part of ourselves that is beyond the ordinary, beyond time and space. It is here that transformation can occur, instantly or in perfect natural timing.

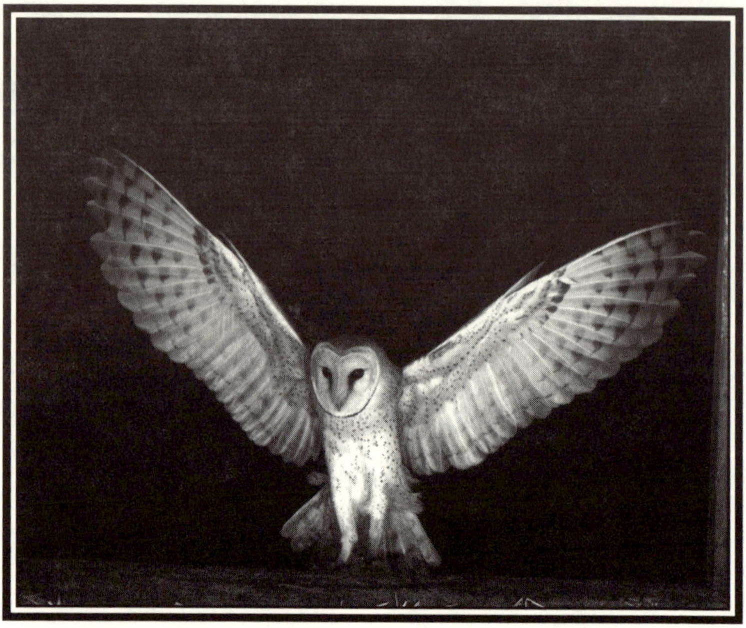

Weaving together opposites creates great strength.

The Gold and Silver Strands

As you begin to move into that place where dreams are made, the voice of the dreams begins to speak. Golden rays filter through the forest. It is easy to see that the light will soon be gone and another world will begin. In the fading golden rays, the little folk begin to peer out cautiously, for it is almost their time. The day fades, the moon begins to rise, and the forest becomes vibrantly alive. Watchful owls nod their approval as, with their silent wings, they move from near to far and back again. The celebration fires are lit, for this is the other world. Children giggle as they flow in and out of invisibility, practicing their newly developing skills. The procession begins with singing and laughter, but with a serious purpose. The little folk weave their way through the forest, and the soft moonlight lights their way. The sounds of their singing prepare the openings to realign. Soon they come to the edge where the sun and moon meet. With joyous celebration, they begin their task of weaving the strands of the sun and moon. As they weave the strands together, things that have been twisted straighten out. And the alignment continues. These glowing strands of gold and silver have many uses. They can be woven into cloth thereby making new habits.

They can be woven into baskets to receive and to carry the natural nourishment of these little folk. These little people are very aware of the other purposes involved in weaving together the strands. Children use these as jump ropes, the girls weave them through their hair, and the fellows use them as belts. Woven together, the strands are very strong. In fact, the little folk also use them as ropes to strengthen things. They may throw one over a tree and use it as a lever to haul something, or to straighten something. But there are more purposes. The little folk instinctively know, that in using those gold and silver strands in many ways and doing these simple chores, the strands work on many different levels. It is fun to watch these little folk discover new uses. Once woven, the strands can reach into those invisible places where the children practice going. As the children practice moving into these new and old places, they can take the strands with them, correcting and adjusting in many different places at once.

As you continue to let go and release that which is no longer necessary, allow the strands to stretch back to the origin. Allow them to do their magic work. You may notice that these strands can be made so fine that you almost cannot see them. Yet they can also be as thick as rope. The little folk collect as much as they need and begin the procession back to their village. Those who have been waiting have prepared a magnificent feast, for they know that these strands reach to the stars and beyond. There is enough for everyone as they weave new garments, and place the strands in their hair. When they gather up a small amount and put the strands in the fire, a very interesting change happens, and they know the exact timing for doing that. The celebration goes on all night. The little folk are very content.

Some of these strands are woven into harps, and when played, make the most amazing music, and the music speaks to all who hear it. The animals join in the singing as they hear this music. For the music from these gold and silver strands affects all who hear it, in the way that is most needed. The first hint of dawn appears at the horizon, and the little folk clear away all traces of their presence, and settle down for their next day's sleep, resting until it is time for them to come out again. While the little folk sleep, the strands continue to work, reaching way back, working their magic far and near, straightening things out. The little folk continue to rest from their joyous night's work, and you can again move from that place and time back to here and now.

The Gold and Silver Strands is about weaving together opposite sides of ourselves to make us stronger—emotions, attitudes, opinions. The story helps us to release old ideas or behaviors making room for the new and creative to emerge from our minds—often when we sleep.

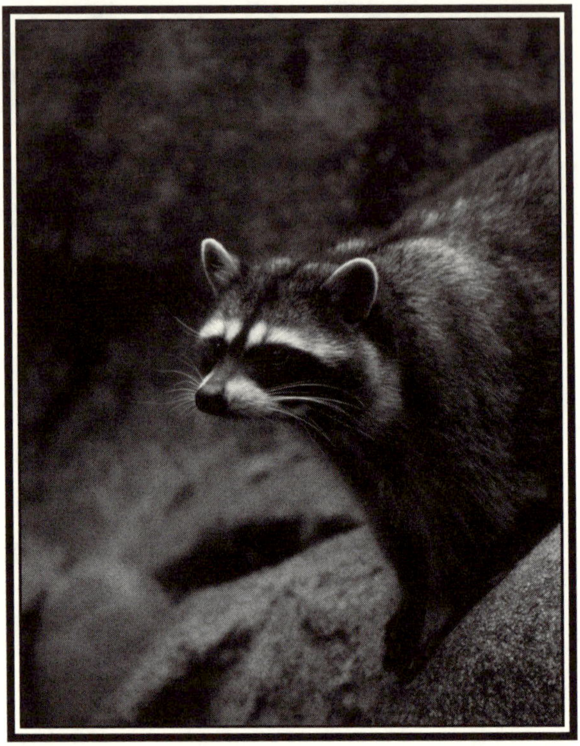

Keep your fears to yourself, but share your courage with others.—Robert Louis Stevenson

The Raccoon Story

THE raccoons were standing on the hill watching the fire sweep through the valley. They felt sad because they knew that a lot of things were being destroyed by the fire, many of their old safe places. They were also happy because they knew that the warning had come in time and their friends and families had all escaped the path of the fire . . . even though some of them got singed a little. They also knew that after the fire was out and the rains came, it would clean things and start new growth. The raccoons had many mixed feelings while they were looking at the fire.

The little raccoon was stamping his foot and having a royal tantrum! He was very angry. The older raccoons nodded approvingly. They understood. The little raccoon stamped around and he threw rocks and he shouted and screamed, but he wasn't hurting anything. The other raccoons didn't try to stop him because they understood. So they watched the fire burn.

Soon the little raccoon, who was still very angry said to one of the older ones, "We've got to find out who started this fire." He knew that it was okay to have fires started by lightening but it was NOT okay to have fires started by monsters.

The raccoons talked among themselves because they all felt the same way. It's just that the little one was expressing it, as he was the loud-mouth of the group. He also had a lot of wisdom for a little one, and expressed what the others didn't. They all decided it @was a good idea, but they didn't want to be rushing off without thinking, they told the little raccoon. They wanted to confer with their friends so they called a meeting. All of the animals of the forest showed up, the hawks and the owls, the eagles and all the birds, the deer, the bunnies and even the snakes. Also the chipmunks, the wolves and the coyotes. They were all very interested in what the raccoons had to say.

This was not the first time there had been trouble. They knew that there were several monsters out there causing the fires. One of the owls had seen them. So the raccoons listened to all the friends and each one had a little piece of information to share with the others. After a while, they came up with a plan. They were going to track down these monsters. The little raccoon was glad because he was still angry.

The older ones and the wise ones knew that they had to be very careful because those monsters were very sneaky. So the raccoons and other animals talked and talked and talked and talked until they all agreed on the plan. Even the little raccoon was impressed. First of all, all the birds went up into the air because they were going to find the monsters. They would do their usual bird things so that the monsters wouldn't notice. Then they would come back and report. It was also decided to put out a call to some of the animals from farther away to help them, like the elephants and the cheetah because he was very fast. They brought in animals from some of the far away lands to help. By this time they were very determined to get those monsters.

It was decided, because the raccoons were already in disguise...you know, because of their masks, that they would lead the group, but they would ride upon the horses. The raccoons aren't really very fast so the horses were more than willing to help. Days later the birds came back. Yes, they had found the monsters planning to destroy other areas. There were three of them. One monster was hiding, one was partly visible and the other one was mostly out in the open. The birds told them where the monsters were. They took with them rocks and clubs and anything that they could think of that they might need. The little raccoon was allowed to go because, well, with his big mouth he insisted on it. After a conference, it was decided that he could go if he paid attention to strict rules. He agreed. He was absolutely delighted that he could go with the older ones. The other younger ones were left safely behind and were being cared for. The little raccoon felt really special because even the little elephant wasn't allowed to go. He made up his mind to be really good so he wouldn't be sent home.

Off they started. The first thing they had to do was to cross the swamp. The elephant helped out by making rafts of logs and the wolf dragged long poles so they could steer. All the other animals gathered things that would be helpful. They made enough rafts for all of them. Of course the one for the elephants had to be larger. They had an owl on each raft because they can see in the dark really well. They sent the bats out ahead with their sonar. Because it was very dark and dismal in the swamp, they started out slowly. They had prepared well. Led by the bat and the owl, they quietly went across the swamp, through the fog. The little raccoon's teeth were chattering a little bit but he hadn't changed his mind and he was still angry.

The animals came to the other side of the swamp, to a new place where none of them had been before. It was the land of the monsters. There were other things that lived in this land and some of them were good and some of them were not. They knew exactly the particular monsters that they were looking for because the birds had seen them. However, there were also various kinds of dragons living here too. Some of the dragons were good and some of them not. Soon they found that they had a few friends over in this land. It was quickly found out that nobody over here liked those three mean monsters they were looking for. In fact, they thought that those monsters shouldn't be in this land at all. I mean, they gave a bad name to monsters. So some of the new creatures helped point the way and gave them maps.

The raccoons in their disguises, led the way. After a time, one of the scouts came back chattering excitedly. The monsters were not far, so they all decided to keep their wits about them and to stop for the night. They built a big fire and made some really good soup. They even sang songs to give them courage. On the outskirts of the circle, some of their new friends were watching and acting as guards. After a while they went to sleep and had dreams of courage and strength. Even the little raccoon was seen to be fighting in his sleep, and growling. They all awakened very, very early and had a quick breakfast. The scouts had gone out and verified the positions of the monsters. The one monster they were not quite positive about, but the birds thought they knew where it was hidden. The other one—well they could see the movement. The third one was out in the open.

They went over their plans again, deciding, changing them a little bit until all were in agreement. The presence of the little raccoon was very good indeed because he reminded all of them of the young ones at home. The young raccoon was put at the end of the group and he didn't object very much, just a little bit. He was given a very important job which was that of the tribe recorder. He took that responsibility very proudly because he knew how sometimes when you get excited in the heat of battles, some things are not remembered. So he knew what an important job it was to be tribe recorder so that everything could be reported accurately to those back home. Indeed, they would make glorious stories.

They started out. The coyotes had shown them all how to sneak up on the monsters without being seen. The raccoons had their masks on. The snakes had shown them how to be quiet. They decided that they were going to attack the monster that was out in the open first. The three monsters were in the same area but they weren't together. Soon, after they came over the rise of a hill, they saw the first monster, a really huge ugly, ugly dragon-looking thing. They all took a deep breath, somebody hollered "Charge!" And they all rushed down the hill, shouting and screaming and hollering, throwing rocks and drawing out their swords. The snakes, going very quickly, acted like ropes and went around the legs. The elephant pushed the monster over and all the animals attacked and attacked. They won the first victory.

The animals were very glad, sort of exhausted and some of them were a little battered and bruised because it had been quite a fight. They decided to rest a while, and again had some more of the good soup. They talked and chattered excitedly, again building up their courage. The lion helped them with that, walking around roaring. Then they were ready for the second bad monster. The plan had to be different because this monster was half hidden. This one was among the trees. They had decided that they were somehow going to circle this monster. They got close enough that they could see what a vile, foul-smelling one it was. This one had longer fangs and teeth than the first one, and was a little more clever. They had planned well and they blocked off the escape route that the monster might take.

This time they sent in the elephants first, and the elephants made as much noise as they could going through the forest. The plan worked because the monster turned to run away and fell into the trap that they had set. The little raccoon recorded it all, as the animals attacked and won the victory over this monster.

They were very, very tired by now and the wise ones decided that it would be foolhardy to go after the monster that was hidden right now. Although they were tired, they retreated back to the hill to a place that was safe, where they could see but couldn't be seen. They allowed themselves plenty of time for rest. The animals were there a couple of days, which gave the little raccoon time to catch up on his recording. He felt better now that two of the bad monsters had been taken care of, and he thought of his little sisters at home and how those monsters couldn't hurt them. So while the bruises healed and they got their strength back, they again sang songs, and getting some details from the little raccoon, made them into wonderful songs.

Then it was time to find the bad monster that was hidden...they had sent their scouts out. The scouts came back and said they had seen tracks. They weren't quite sure where this one was, but they had seen the tracks, which seemed to lead over to the place where there were rocks, big rocks. Someone guessed that this monster was in a cave. They animals thought and they thought and they thought and they decided it would be much better if they could get the monster out of the cave. Soon they came up with a plan, a very clever plan. They sent the scouts out again to make sure of some details and to get accurate maps. The scouts came back and gave them the information they needed.

The plan was very clever indeed. First, the horses went on top of what they knew was the cave, and they reared and whinnied. The horses trampling on the roof of rocks made a horrendous thundering noise. The clever little monkeys had dropped fireballs down the air vent to the cave and soon the smoke started to roll out of the entrance of the cave. The other animals were hiding nearby, waiting. Soon, from in the cave, they heard the most awful bellowing. And they waited. Now the elephants joined the horses in making noise. Straw was stuffed down the air vent to make more smoke. Still they waited. The bellowing continued. Soon, with a great roar, the monster came running out of the cave and all of the animals attacked. Some of them blocked off the entrance of the cave so the monster couldn't get back in. Some of them tripped him. Some of them poked his eyes so he couldn't see. They attacked as hard as they could because he was the sneakiest, biggest and the most mean and violent of all. He almost destroyed their entire land and all who lived there.

After a long hard battle, the animals won. They were almost too exhausted to celebrate. However, they built a big fire and made a feast. All the animals of the new land, including the good monsters, celebrated too. They all sang and danced. After the feast, they all went to the water pool. You can imagine, they were very dirty. They had been fighting and had been gone from home a long time. They romped and played in the water. Some of them played peek-a-boo behind the waterfall, and the elephants made other waterfalls by squirting water out of their trunks. Even the ones who were a little afraid of water were helped by the others. They had a grand time in the water.

Now it was time to go home. They had all taken a piece of the monster's fur and made headbands and decorations. The coyote had a piece of fur tied onto his tail. They started their procession back home. The other creatures of monster-land cheered them as they passed by. On the road, they met an elder dragon who said to one of the wise ones, "Come with me, there's something I've been guarding for a very long time that I want to share because you have made this land of ours safe for us too, you know." So the elder dragon led the wise one deep into a secret cave. There were many, many treasures in that cave. There were stacks and stacks of pearls and gems of all kinds. There were many rooms of different treasures and the old dragon said, "Please take some of these. Take them for each of the animals as a token of our thanks." The wise one felt very honored and promised the elder dragon to keep the secret of the cave. The dragon nodded because he already knew that this wise one had integrity and was very honorable.

The rest of the animals were astounded at the beauty of the treasures. They promised to visit back and forth so they could learn about each other's lands and customs. They each thought the other was unusual and so looked forward to visiting. "There is another way back that is a short cut," said the elder dragon. "I will show you where it is." He pointed off in the distance and there was a bridge.

"Go over that bridge," the elder dragon said, "and that way you won't have to go back through the swamp." They were most grateful and off they went, carrying banners and flags and all kinds of things, in a procession of victory. Waving to their new-found friends, they went over the bridge. Sure enough, it was a short cut. Now those that had been left at home heard the noise and began to smile for they could tell this was the noise of victory. They could hear the noise from far off so they got busy preparing a welcome celebration, fixing many different foods, not forgetting anyone for some of the animals had unusual tastes. They made special dishes for all of them.

Well, the welcome home feast was absolutely incredible. Even the little raccoon, who had been appointed the tribe recorder, was a hero. They had a marvelous celebration, thanking everyone. They gave great speeches and honored each other. The wise ones ended with speeches reminding all that peace was the most important thing and that fighting was only for defending land and families.

The Raccoon Story helps us to deal with anger and general acceptance of feelings, including grief. The story shows the value of planning and preparation, teamwork, courage in facing fears and 'monsters'. It focuses on the values of listening, being open to ideas, gratitude, integrity and responsibility. The story encourages taking action and acknowledging and accepting differences as we connect with others. This story is also helps in trusting our own wisdom.

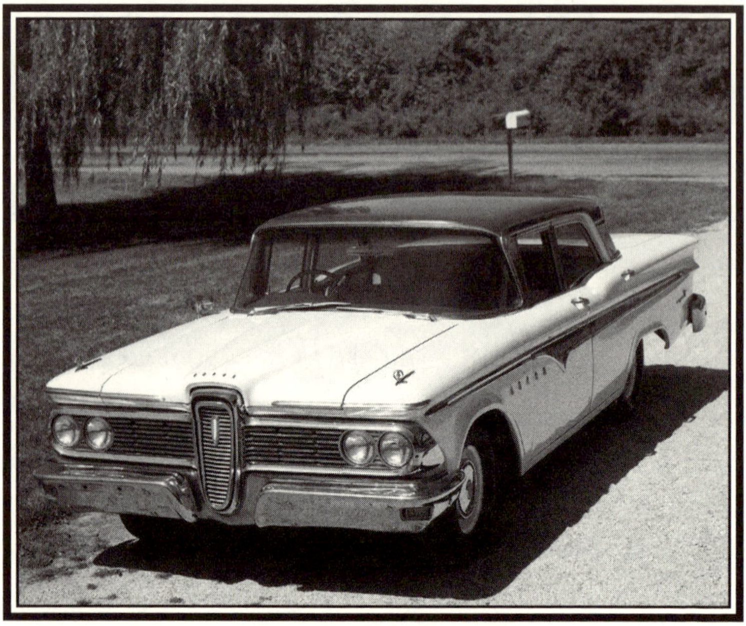

To face despair and not give in to it, that's courage.

—Ted Koppel

THE CAR

THE car slowed to a stop at the side of the road to look at the view. He loved looking at nature. He turned off his motor so that he could hear the trickling sound of the water in the little stream. He enjoyed watching the way the water went over and around the rocks as it made its relaxing sound. Looking up, he noticed the vibrant colors of the wildflowers mixed in with the green grass in the meadow. A gentle breeze sang through the trees causing the leaves to dance and the young trees to sway. The car liked the pine trees the best because they smelled so good. No matter how he felt, looking at nature made him feel better.

The car sighed, partly from contentment, partly because he was hurting. He was no longer young and the accidents over the years had left him with some damage. Most of the accidents had been minor, but the last accident where the truck had gone through the stop sign and hit him, had caused him to be out of alignment and even his back wheels ached. He had made some poor choices through the years which further damaged him. The car had become discouraged. He had thought of giving up and going to the scrap yard, but he decided not to. He really loved the world, the animals and most of the people. He didn't even mind hauling heavy boxes from one place to another. He enjoyed working and helping others.

After one last look at the blue sky with its soft, white clouds, he started his engine and continued on his way. His engine wasn't working well and was making a strange sound. Over the years, he had repairs in many different garages. Some of the repairs had been good, some had made things worse but the car kept moving on, doing his jobs, having his adventures. The car was concerned that he was now beyond repair. He had many different things wrong with him and was feeling hopeless.

The car wasn't on a job at the moment. He was going on a pleasure trip, driving wherever he wanted and stopping when he was tired. He didn't have a particular destination in mind but was simply exploring. He saw a sign that said Hopeville, 5 miles. *I've never been there,* he thought to himself. *I think I will look it over.* He turned onto the country road leading to Hopeville, noticing there were gently rolling hills ahead. In the distance, he saw someone walking in the road . As the car came closer he wondered if the person wanted a ride. The car liked to give rides because he got to meet many different people. The name on the back of the person's blue coveralls said Angela's Car Service. The car noticed she had her hair tucked up under a ball cap.

"Hello," said the car, "would you like a ride?" She turned toward him and he noticed the name Angel above her pocket—short for Angela, he guessed.

"Thank you," said Angel. "That would be great."

The door sagged as she opened it. She climbed in and tugged the door so that it closed. The car noticed there was a soft glow about her.

Angel made no mention of the sagging seat or the peeling dashboard, weathered by the sun. Angel asked questions about the unusual noises the car made, his pains, his complaints. She listened carefully to his answers about what the car thought was wrong with him. She asked him about his life and the car responded easily, talking to her as he had never talked to anyone else. It was interesting how easy she was to talk to, thought the car.

"You are very kind," said Angel, "and have helped many people in your life." The car acknowledged what she said and then humbly said, "But there were things in my life that I did wrong and I'm not proud of them."

"Did you learn from your experiences?" Angel asked.

"I sure hope so," sighed the car. "I just want to be kind and help where I can—and that isn't very much anymore," he said sadly. It was amazing to note how much was accomplished as they drove those final 2 miles to Hopeville. Almost as if they had stepped outside of time.

Hopeville was a charming small town with a magical feel. The buildings wore flower boxes with brightly colored flowers facing tree-lined streets. There was an old fashioned town clock, too. Angel pointed down the street. "That's my place," she said. The car limped down the street and pulled into the driveway of Angela's Car Service. As Angel shoved the door open and got out, she faced the car and said, "I want to help you if you are willing. Right now it would be helpful to you to have some water." The car wondered how she knew that and gratefully accepted the water. He had been almost dry. "Are you willing to accept my help?" Angel asked. An unusual question thought the car. "I'm not sure I can be helped, but yes, I'm willing." Angel guided the car over to a service bay and said, "First it is important for you to rest. We will start tomorrow."

The car sighed, for he was very tired and was grateful for the opportunity to rest. It was almost as if Angel could read his mind. He faced the street, watching the town for a short time, then slept soundly.

Angel appeared early the next morning, and this time she wore violet coveralls. "Good morning," she said to the car, "did you sleep well?"

"Surprisingly, yes," replied the car.

Angel looked intensely at the car, her eyes seeing far more than the exterior. Quietly she walked all around the car, stopping in some places before moving on. The car felt a little strange because somehow he knew she was looking all the way through him.

"Car, I work very differently than any mechanic you've had before. First we have to work on your attitude." The car felt surprised. "Your attitude can help or interfere," she said. Coming close to him, she placed her hands on his hood. The glow coming from her was much stronger now. Her hands felt warm, almost hot, but comforting. The car felt himself relaxing against her touch. What a wonderful feeling he thought. He felt it in many places. A strong but slight vibration coursed through his entire being, from his front bumper to the back. Angel stayed there a long time. The car noticed a very small feeling of hope begin. Finally, Angel lifted her hands and said, "Well?" The car looked at her thoughtfully and nodded and smiled.

Angel told him that he was to remember that feeling. "You can do that yourself. You just need to practice." The car was skeptical but agreed to give it a try. Next Angel lifted the car's hood and stared inside. The car had been correct, it was a mess, with many things needing to be fixed. Then she hoisted the car up in the air. The back axle was bent and the entire structure was out of alignment. She lowered the car back down and looked at him. "I admire you, car," she said. "I admire that you have been able to keep going as long as you have." Although she had not yet examined the engine, she knew there was trouble there also.

Angel began to glow more as she spoke with him. She seemed to glide as she walked around the car. "Your part in this is very important," she told the car. She explained that he needed to visualize everything working well. "It's been so long that I'm not sure I know how to do that."

"Use your imagination. A little at a time if you need to. Maybe you can remember how it felt a long time ago when you were healthier. Or maybe you can pretend you are like another car you've seen that works well. Do this every day. More than once a day is better. It's a beginning and you need to be persistent. I know you know how." The car felt Angel's faith in him. A welcome jolt of energy coursed through him.

Angel picked up some tools and went to work under the hood, fixing connections, rewiring, strengthening weak parts, adjusting the timing, putting it into its perfect rhythm. Again the car had the sense of being outside of time. The car tried to remember the feeling of relaxation he had experienced earlier, then began to imagine his tires against the asphalt rolling on a smooth road feeling all its parts working together as fine tuned as he wanted to be. It wasn't easy but he did his best because he promised himself that he would do his part as she asked.

After a while, Angel stopped work. "It's time you rested now," she said. "Much work is done when you don't notice. You might be surprised how much healing can occur automatically, once adjustments are put into motion." She gave him more water and told him she would see him in the morning.

The car again rested well, which he considered a miracle. Angel appeared the next morning in gold coveralls and asked how he was doing. "I don't seem to be hurting as much," said the car.

"I want you to drive out to the highway and then come back," she said. The car started out of the garage, drove to the end of Hopeville and down the road toward the highway, then back to the garage. Angel looked at him and the car knew she wanted a report. He had paid attention and told her he felt stronger, his timing was good, the pain was less, and he felt straighter. Angel's glow increased and she again walked around the car looking deep into him. As she stopped in front of him she said, "Things are beginning to change. You need to think about the anger you have felt and be willing to release it. That includes anger at yourself. You need to keep working on letting go of fear. You must be grateful for what you have. That's an important one. Gratitude is like the fertilizer in a garden. It helps good things grow. You need to love what and how you are. Work on these every day. Remember to have a lot of water and make sure you get the right fuel and oil. I know helping others is important to you, so continue to do what you can. It makes you happy. It's time for you to continue on your journey." The car was sad to think of leaving. Angel put her hand on his hood and again the car felt warm and relaxed and hopeful. "Some things take time. Don't get discouraged. You must continue to work on yourself, accepting and loving the way you are now. Focus on every moment.

You will know when it is time to come back again. You may return at any time. Expect miracles and have fun in your adventures. Remember the love and peace you feel from me. It is everywhere in the world."

The car was indeed grateful, and peaceful too. As he continued on his journey he knew how blessed he was and radiated love to the wildflowers, the trees, the animals and the people he met, helping where he could, determined to heal as much as possible.

The Car story helps to give hope when someone needs it. This story is mostly for people with chronic or multiple problems. It assists in accessing our own intuition and wisdom while addressing emotions which might be blocking healing or change. It shows the importance of visualization and of helping others.

The spiritual life does not remove us from the world but leads us deeper into it.

—Henri J. M. Novwen

PART II

NAVIGATING THE COLORS—MEDITATIONS

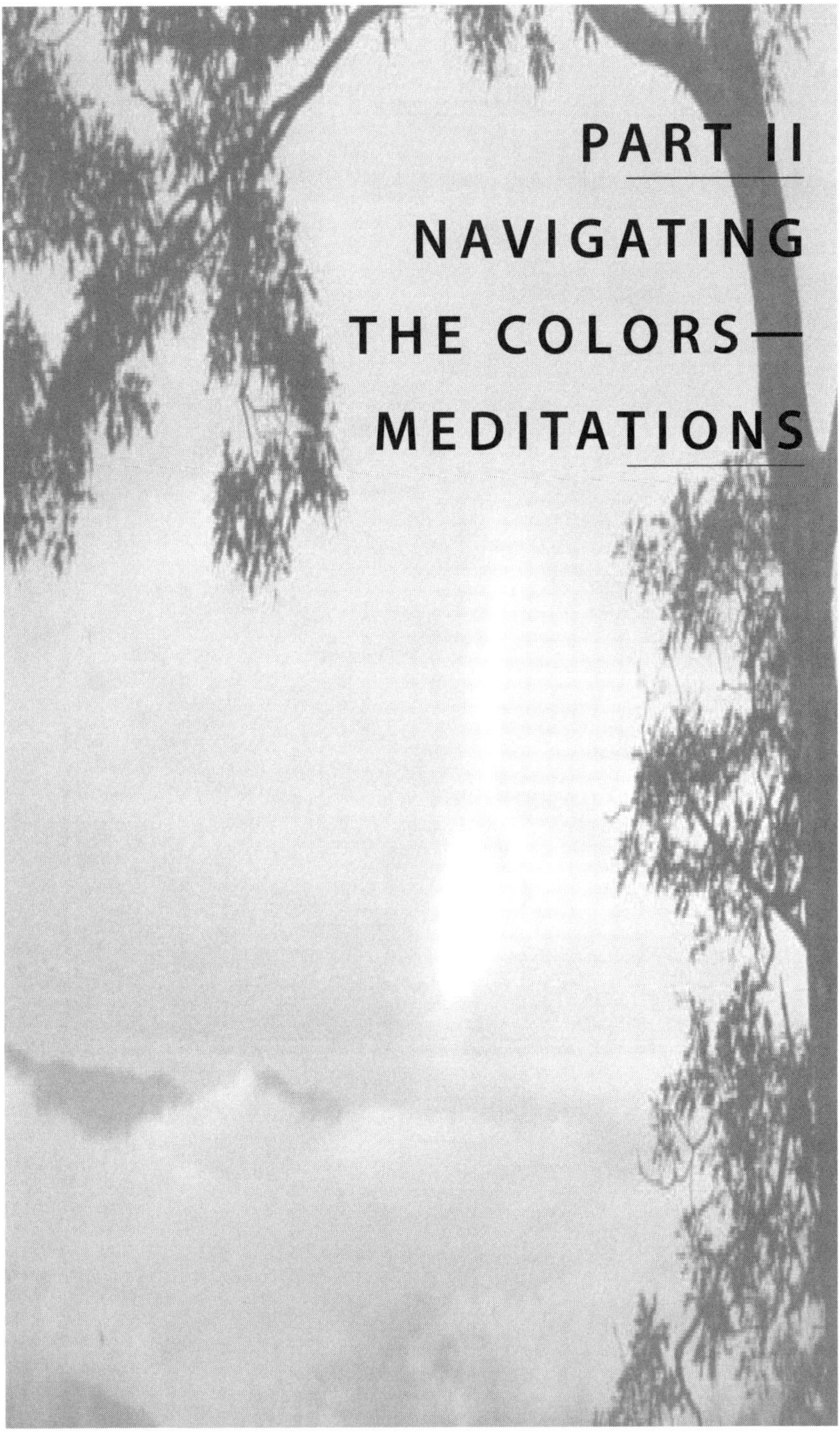

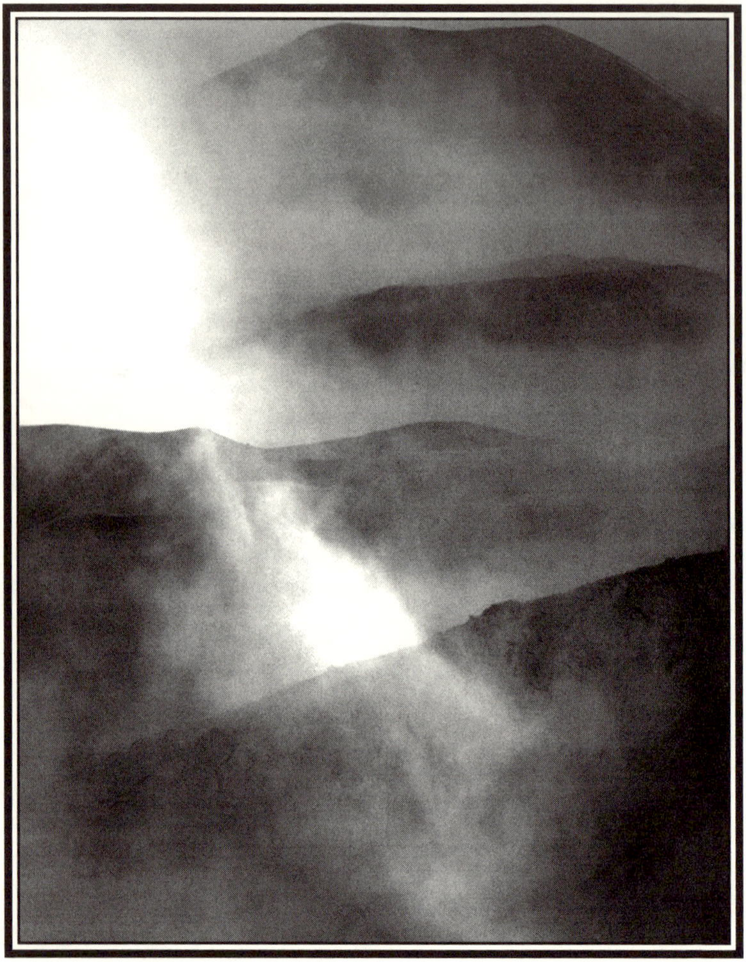

In Between the Mist

IN the aftermath of a warm summer's rain, the air holds a coolness and a freshness. The moisture that remains forms a mist that one cannot see. Yet the skin can drink in that cool, refreshing water, for it is in such a fine form that the skin can absorb it easily. You drift into that fine summer mist, and it seems you pass between particles that are very fine. That space is refreshing. Your body begins to feel much more at ease as its moisture balance is re-established. The light catches those unseen particles and the tiniest ribbons of colors weave themselves in and out of the dew drops. You continue on this journey as if you are walking in a rainbow forest. Objects, people and forms of many varieties begin to take shape as you move through a kaleidoscope of mist and colors. Notice the shapes that take form. The journey through the spaces can be as exciting as the journey through the forms. It is interesting to see the light vary in intensity from light to dark to light. Like that space at the edge of day and night and night to day, there is something special about that transition.

Drifting deeper into the shadows and into the rainbow shadows, it's as if a whole other world becomes visible. You may be aware of the comforting presence of others walking very close to you, for there are those who live in this time and space and who know it very well. They are the guides to those worlds that lie between worlds. Allow yourself to be guided through the dimensions of the in-between. You can be aware that all information that you are collecting is safe and secure in your memory banks, to which you will have easy access. It is not surprising that this space feels familiar. Experiences often have no words. Yet they can be recreated using combinations of elements. As you continue to release that creative energy, many new creations can emerge. They may be creations of words, colors, or shapes. Remember the softness of the unseen mist and how it is possible to see what others do not see. It is possible to be in that space between those microscopic drops of water even as they, in turn, travel on the winds of time. There is an answer to every riddle, and an answer to every question as you continue to allow yourself to use the energy of creation. Now you begin to travel back. Notice the sounds as you move through those spaces in the mist, feeling the ever-comforting moisture. Re-entering the ribbon rainbows, move through those ribbons of color, and back into the fullness of here and now.

Moving from Here to There

THERE are times when it gets very, very dark and we can't see. There are also times when it gets very dark and we can't feel or hear. It would be easy to think, at those times, that the darkness is all that there is. But that is not so. At those times, in the darkness, where you can't see or feel or hear, there is something that can be activated—something that has been dormant for a long time. It is interesting, when you know how, to move instantaneously out of the darkness. And you do know how. When that happens, it's as though you are looking down on a tar pit. When you are looking down, you may think, *how did I ever exist in that tar pit*—but you did. And you may be thinking, *how did I get out*—but you did, for many things are there, even though we do not see them. There are many ways and paths, although we do not hear or feel them. There is a bridge that connects it all. When you are in the darkness, it is hard to see the bridge. But if you know that there might be a bridge, somehow with that extra knowledge, you can find it. How freeing it is to be able to pass to that place where everything feels so good, where you are free of everything that had been limiting. When you are on this other side, there is much more understanding of why you went into the darkness in the first place.

Occasionally you know that you may need to dip back into that darkness for additional understanding. But now that you know where the bridge is . . . . This new place is beyond anything that you can imagine. It feels like the glowing sun. It smells like the fresh land after a cleansing rain. It sounds like laughter or the cooing noises that a happy baby makes. It also feels like the strength of the lion. This is a very different place, and you can find it. You know how a bat can find its way, even though it cannot see? This bat is very accurate. It's like that. You know how warm the ground feels when you are lying down in a meadow in the summer, with that great aroma? It's like that. You know the endurance the horse shows as he runs and runs and runs? It's like that. You know how it feels to the eagle, simply to rest on the currents of the wind? It's like that. You know how soft a little kitten feels? Or the velvety feel of flower petals? It's like that. If you can remember how good it feels to take a deep breath on a clear, crisp day when the air is clear, you can remember how this place feels, and it's like that. It is also like the colors of the rainbow when they all are balanced in line and fit together. The rainbows always seem to awaken that which needs to be awakened. The rainbow can carry you where you need to go. Remember the cool mountain stream, that happily bubbles along making its own path to where it needs to go? It's like that. It has the beauty of all the stars and the comfort of moonlight. Somehow, it is with all these sensations that when you least expect it, the miracles appear. It can be quite amusing when you realize that they are always there. The child knows as he runs through the grass with his hands open to catch the rainbows.

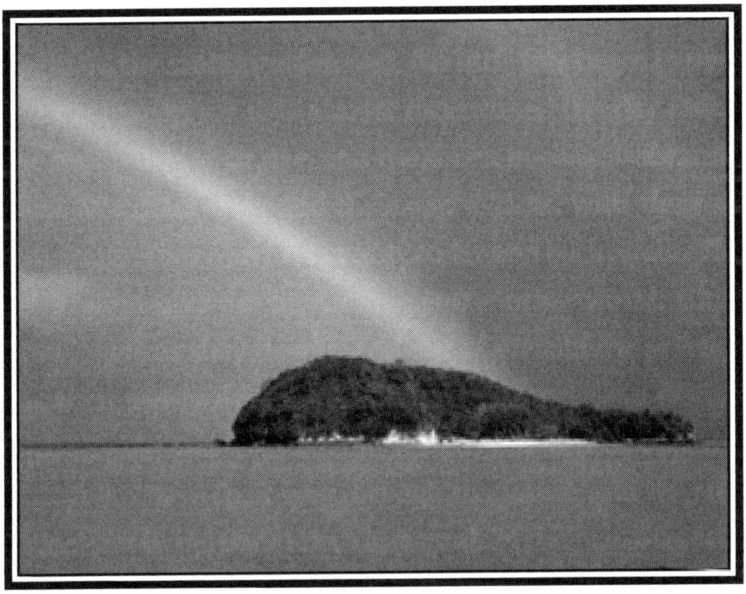

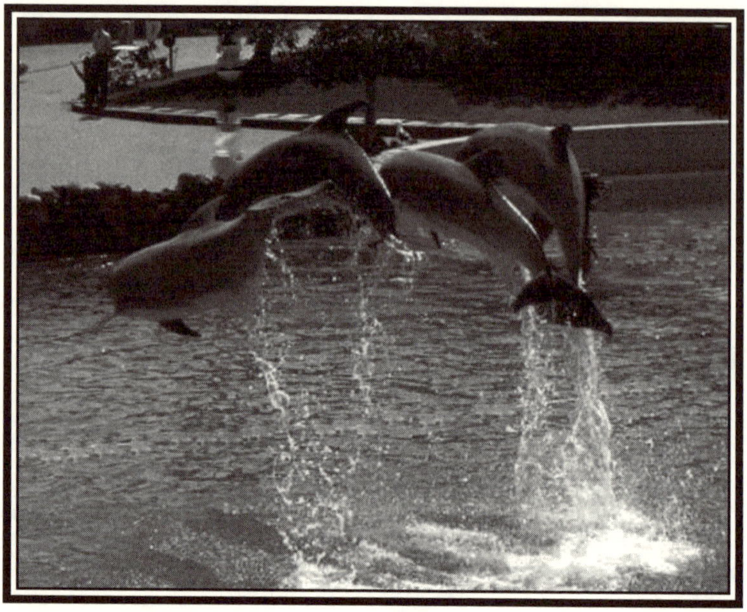

Dolphins

I AM reminded even now of that seemingly gentle movement the dolphin makes as it propels itself through the water. It's as if there is no resistance as its body moves, in a way almost to suggest that that neither one touches the other, yet its movement is rhythmic and smooth. The water feels its presence as directed by nature. The sound of its graceful body plays a melody that you can hear when you listen. There may be the whoosh and the splash of the physical sound, yet behind those sounds plays a sometimes even louder dolphin melody. The dolphin for its size, travels so easily, with rhythm, grace, speed, and with an instinct that is strong and clear. When a dolphin speaks sounds that man has interpreted, man and dolphin bridge a truly remarkable link. Their affinity for one another is well known. Such a wonderful sight, to watch a dolphin as he comes to the surface and goes down again—whoosh. The sea about him often changes colors from deep blue to blue-green and sometimes green. The dolphins are very playful. There is something about watching them move that is hypnotic and soothing, as if we are able to ride the crest of Mother Nature simply by watching their precise movements. Watching schools of dolphins multiplies the delight. I think it would be fun to ride on top of one, allowing yourself to travel with the dolphins.

The sounds are magnificent. While you're riding, you don't want to miss a thing. It's easy to be totally with that experience. When you ride, there is nothing else you'd rather be doing, nothing else on your mind. It is pure pleasure during the times that you ride the dolphin. It might be fun, too, to swim with the dolphins.

A dolphin might prove to be a most interesting guide as you tour the ocean's wonderland. It might be fun too, to see the ocean through a dolphin's eyes. There are other creatures to notice. It is interesting to notice the currents in the waters that the dolphins travel, for they can travel great distances in a day's time. If dolphins would play human games, I wonder what games they would choose to play. If humans were to choose dolphin games, I wonder which ones they would choose.

Watching the dolphins, swimming with the dolphins, riding the dolphins—such wonderful choices, each a possibility. Experiencing each one at its right time and place can be most fulfilling. You can watch the dolphins from a platform, from the shore, from a boat or an airplane, or even a helicopter. It's fun to know you can choose one on one day, fully experience it, then choose a different method another day and fully experience it. The dolphins continue their dance of the ages. Their shiny, water-covered skin comes to the surface, and on sunny days the rays catch that surface, reflecting beautiful pictures. It is almost as if they are not real. Sometimes it seems as if they are standing still—yet they can be moving at a very fast speed. They are beautiful animals: intelligent and able to communicate more easily than other animals. There is something very snuggly about them, as though you want to be close to them. Many books are written about dolphins, their habits and abilities and many pictures have been taken of these creatures, and yet I wonder if we will ever really know everything there is to know about them, their mystery, their enchantment, their intrigue. It truly is a wondrous time, spending the day with the dolphins.

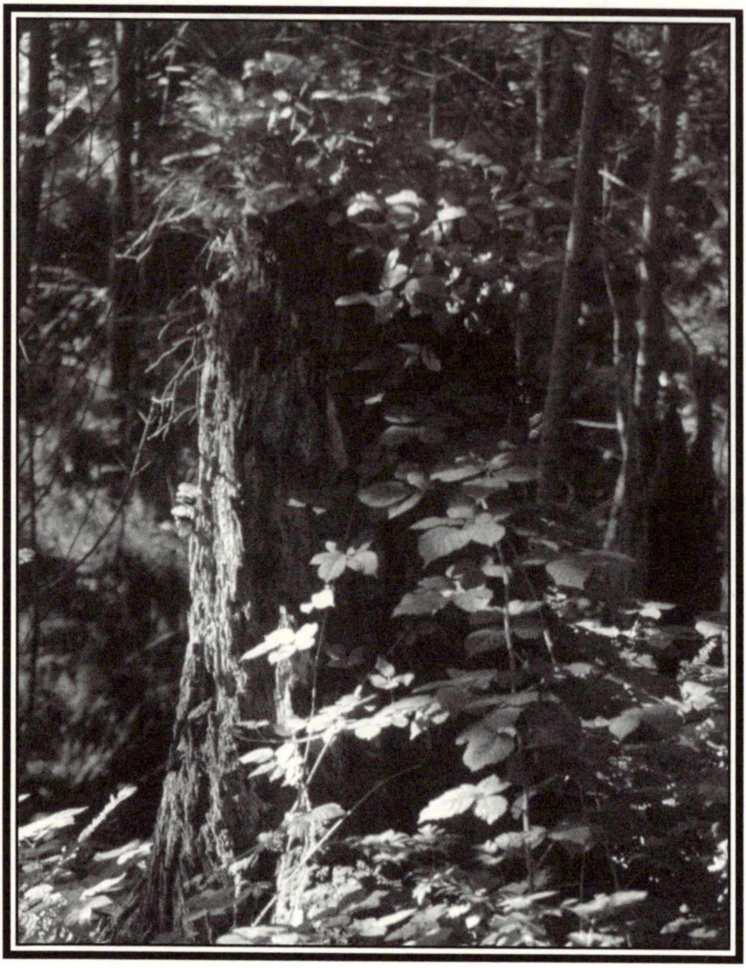

Shifting Images

YOU begin to relax, and you may find yourself remembering the layers of the sweet-smelling clothes hanging in the sun on a clothesline. It is comforting to get lost in that marvelous, fresh smell. There's something about the sun and the wind that combines to create that wonderful aroma. The coolness of the clothes brushing on your skin adds another sensation. Notice how comfortable you feel walking through those clothes, allowing yourself to get lost in the fresh clean smell. It is like, but different from being wrapped up in flannel or being in a tree. There are times when things seem the same when they're not and other times things seem different when they're not. Remember that feeling of freshness, warmth and coziness, sitting in front of a fire after you've had a nice warm bath, and are wrapped in flannel. It's amazing how this feeling can be taken anywhere you want, even sitting on a rock in the forest. While sitting on that rock, feeling how solid that rock is, it's almost the same as but different from sitting in the tree and feeling how solid the tree is. The smell in the forest—notice that smell and how it wraps around you almost like the smell of the clothes, the smell of the fire, different, but somewhat the same, too. It's funny to think that you can be on a rock in the forest and at the same time be in the clothes and in front of the fire, but you can. Then, of course, there's the sound of the stream. Even that has a fresh smell and a marvelous feel. It's fun to hear the stream without looking and sometimes it's fun to look in the stream and get lost in it, like you got lost in the clothes or lost in the trees. Of course you are not lost at all. You are really found. Notice how freely that water flows. Notice how easily the water flows over and around anything that is in its way. The sound—how soothing is the sound of the water. It's not unlike the sound of the quiet in the forest or the sound of the wind through the clothes on the line, or the sound of the wind through the trees. Again, how easily you can be in more than one place at once. For sitting in the tree, feeling the bark, the sturdiness of the tree, the freedom at the same time, smelling that wonderful tree smell, you can also be among the clothes, in the forest or by the stream. Indeed it is possible to be in more than one place at once, and most people don't know that. When looking at a rainbow, those beautiful colors, some people think that the rainbow connects the sky to the earth. But does it not also connect the earth to the sky? It's fascinating to see which color you feel like being in at any given moment. How naturally you gravitate to the one you need. Sometimes it seems that the rainbow is in all things. If you cannot see it you can at least feel it. Sometimes you can see it in the stream. Can't you also feel it in the clothes, or in the forest or in the trees?

Think about the birds. Birds are very wise, and they know how to see things from an entirely different perspective. If you take a trip with a bird, you will notice how easy it is to see from different perspectives. And yet, with that wonderful free feeling of soaring with the bird, can you not also remember and be again in more than one place at once, and feel yourself sitting on a rock in the forest, or lying down by the stream, or being in a tree. How easily and quickly the shift can occur. It's almost as if you are seeing things in different light. Notice the change between the same scenes seen in the sunlight, and seen in the moonlight. It is easy to see things in a different light. It can be really fun. Soaring with that bird, you may find a clear pool of water somewhere and as you look at that pool from above, you notice something coming to the surface. As you and your bird friend swoop down for a closer look, bubbles rise from deep within, gently floating to the surface and popping. How interesting it must be from the perspective of the fish who can follow that bubble from the depths all the way to the surface where it pops and releases. It is curious to wonder what these bubbles are releasing. Notice the ease with which they gently float to the surface and pop. The water then joins the rest of the water in a very natural way. It is very soothing to feel the water on your skin. It can be amusing to wrap yourself around the bubble, make yourself its size and go for a ride as it gently goes to the surface. If you look closely, there is the rainbow again in the bubble. You can become very playful. How easily things that were uncomfortable become comfortable, just like the rock, the tree, the stream, sitting in front of the fire, floating up with the bubble and the free soaring with the bird. Notice also how you can control the scenes you are seeing. You can be in them all, or watch them all. It is easy to control this in any way you choose. Notice how all the scenes have the quality of soothing comfort, wrapped in flannel by the fire, hearing that wonderful crackling noise, feeling that rock beneath you in the forest, pretending you are a fish or a dolphin, and sure, you can imagine it's in a pool and feel just as comfortable, as sitting in a tree hearing the wind, or walking among the clothes that have been freshly washed, feeling the warmth of the sun and coolness of the clothes, or lying by the stream. Notice how easy it is to go to any or all of these places instantaneously. Because, of course you know the secret of being in more than one place at once. That's right, feeling very relaxed. It is so nice to know that healings can come in many, many ways and can be applied to children of all ages. As you are floating around with your bird, notice how sometimes when you see the clouds they may look very concentrated to you. But it doesn't take much to disperse them with the wind, or the sun can do magic and disperse that which was concentrated, into little fine wisps which float away in the breeze. And the ever-present rainbow is still there to connect the earth with the sky.

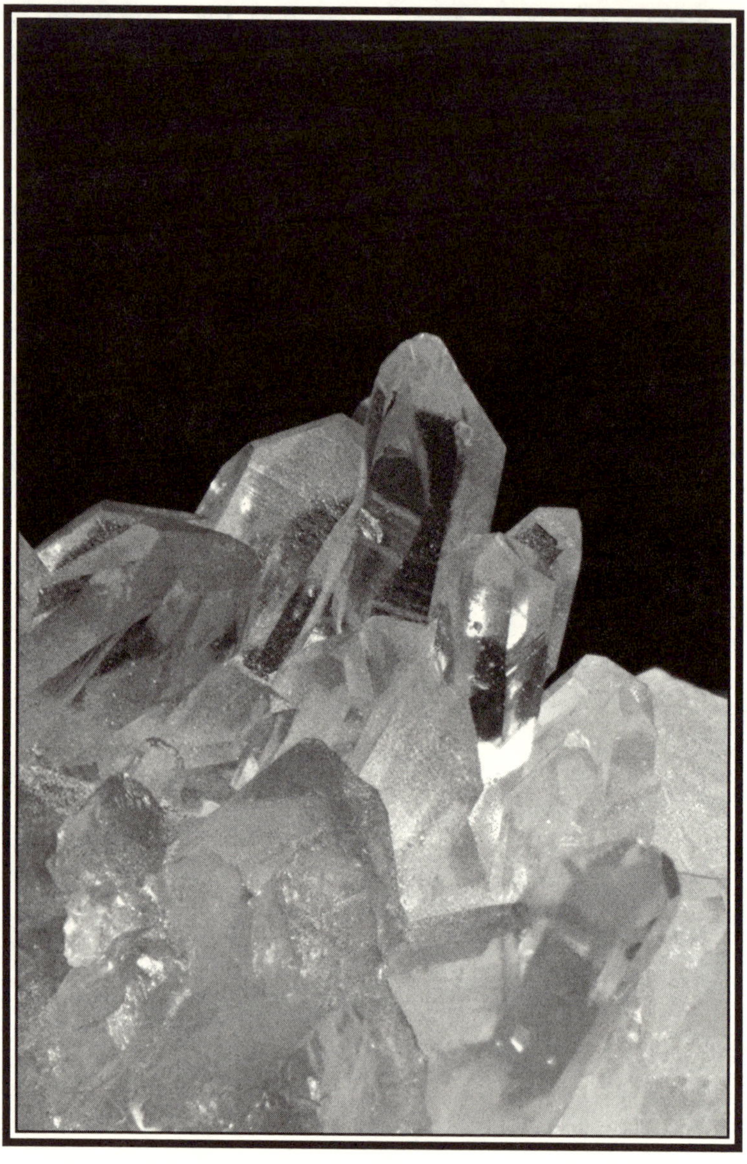

©Jubal Harshaw

The World of Crystals

THE gentle sounds that surround you continue to play their own special melody, and you can begin to feel yourself traveling. It is fun to notice the method you have chosen to travel, and it may be a method that you cannot quite identify in terms in how you have related to travel in the past. Notice how the gentle currents of nature provide wonderful assistance. You may notice a movement when you adjust and re-adjust to the speed of the medium through which you are traveling. The movements of one substance to another can be warm and comforting. The sounds of far-away lands beckon as you accelerate toward your destination. The sights, the sounds, and smells all merge in a whirlwind of experience. As you change from one speed to another, there may be a burst of color or an unusual sound or feeling. You find yourself entering a crystal world, the likes you have never seen. You are familiar with the crystals of water and ice and you are familiar with the crystals of the earth. These crystals are similar but very different. The energy in this place is soft and comforting as if certain parts of yourself have finally connected with an energy that speaks to them. The crystals seem to grow before your eyes, as their shape and formation are in motion. The feel of these crystals is wonderful. Much like the energy they convey, to touch them is to touch softness, and yet it might not seem so. They appear to be a material that takes a definite form. It is pleasant to run your hands up one side and down the other of any particular crystal that intrigues you. Sometimes you can see crystals within the crystal. There are the most interesting combinations of shapes, and you may color these crystals any color you want. The colors add a different feel, a different texture. and if you listen carefully, a different sound. It seems as if you could walk right through these colored crystal structures. Light that appears to arrive from a far distant place adds its own magic to the colors you have chosen. As you continue to let go and hold on. Holding on and yet allowing yourself to be carried away by the color, the light, the sound, the feel. You can feel it all together, and you can feel it separately. You can rearrange the crystals, and change their positions for they are willing to serve, as their true nature remains intact in spite of their color or where they are placed. It is fun to hold on to the crystals, and it is fun to let them go. In some crystals you may find words or combination of words familiar to you now, or familiar to you from before. Plants and flowers grow among these crystals. You can play the crystals to make beautiful melodies. This crystal city travels and you may continue to travel with it, or travel in your own direction. It is truly amazing what one can see with one's heart as the boundaries between worlds seem to melt away. How at home you feel in this ever-changing universe no matter where you go, no matter what you choose to experience.

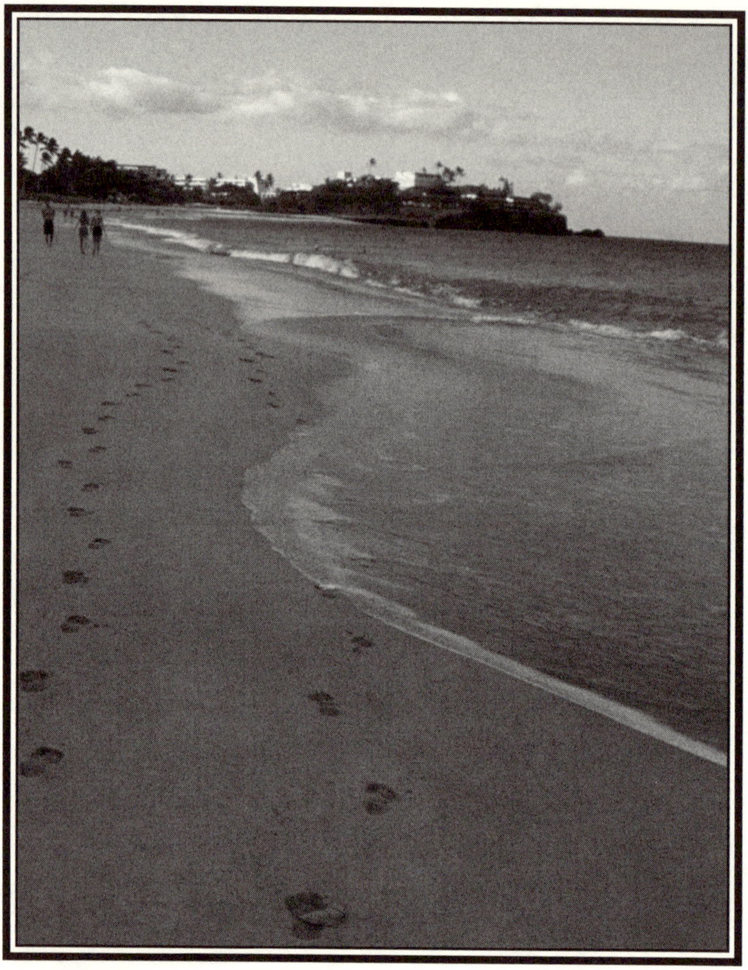

The Sands of Time

As you allow yourself to drift with the winds of time, and with the sands of time, it is fun to remember those temperate days at the beach, walking barefoot in the sand. As you near the water, the sand becomes moist. As you move away from the water it becomes dry and separates more easily. It is fun to run and skip, and to let the water run up over your feet. It's fun, too, to take an object, like a piece of wood that has drifted up on the beach, to write or draw in the sand. There is something about being in that sand. It brings the past to the present and beyond. The water erases the footprints, the names, the messages in the sand. Sometimes immediately, sometimes only as the tide comes in. If you've ever experienced a red tide in the warm summer evening, there's something magical about the phosphorescent light in the water. Watching it, or swimming in it can be an experience, almost as if small pieces of stars have fallen to the earth and have magnetized themselves together. It is beautiful to watch the tops of the waves glisten and shine as they rise and fall. If you have been at the ocean in a full moon when the grunion have run, there is something magical about the dance of these small living sea creatures as they follow their natural instincts, and deposit their eggs in the moonlight above the ocean. On a warm evening the sight may be as close to paradise as can be found here on earth. Allow yourself to be carried still further inside the sands of time. Did you ever make sand candles? Did you paint with sand? Do you walk among the tide pools and notice the movement of tiny sea life, plants and animals? In far away places, you can smell the fragrant blossoms of plants that grow near the shore. Did you sit on the beach on a warm day, look at the sky, and notice the airplanes that write their messages against the deep blue? Sometimes airplanes carry their messages behind them on banners. When those airplanes are writing their messages in the sky, they may seem upside down or backwards or seem to go in a different direction from where you are sitting. You need to tilt your head or stand on your head to figure out what they are spelling. It is fun. Words and letters show themselves for a short time, then are dissipated by the atmosphere, awaiting new messages, new letters, new words. There is always so much going on at the beach. In summer it is fun to watch the parade of bathers walking back and forth, running into the water and back to shore, talking to each other, listening to the radio, eating lunch or turning from side to side to bathe in the rays of the sun. The human animal comes in so many varieties—different combinations of hair, skin, eyes, and expressions. It is fun to see the many different ways in which their parts are assembled and look so different. Even the bathing suits, the colors, the different styles on males, females and children. It's fun too to watch the games that go on, the frisbees as they are thrown in the air. Those who are adept can spin them on their fingers and hands and catch them behind their backs. It is amazing what they can do with a small piece of plastic. Paddle tennis and other games and entertainment come to the beach. In some places, during summer heat, you can walk to the snack stand with all sorts of wonderful goodies, cold things, gooey things, crispy things. Being outdoors seems to liven the senses. As the day at the beach begins to connect with the night and people pack up to return to their homes, there's a certain feeling, a little like the feeling that hangs in the stadium after a big game with much cheering, as if the impression of the day's activities hangs there reaching for the last few moments of the day. Colors change along the horizon. A gentle breeze stirs and moves across the sand and the ocean. It is very peaceful, a good time and place to be with the universe and yourself. It is hard to turn and leave. A magnetic something draws the soul there until the last bit of sunlight is gone. You continue to drift with the sands of time. Reach in, connect with, and pull out everything you need. Things come together as you remember there are so many different ways to write—many different mediums to use, many different colors, many different words and combinations. It is as if the sun proposes to the earth each morning. With the dawning of this new day, you can allow yourself to drift again back with sands of time to this place, here and now.

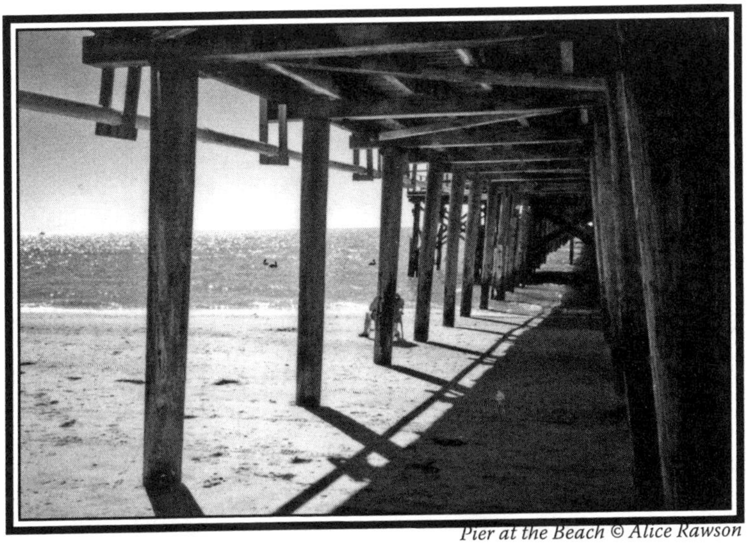

Pier at the Beach © Alice Rawson

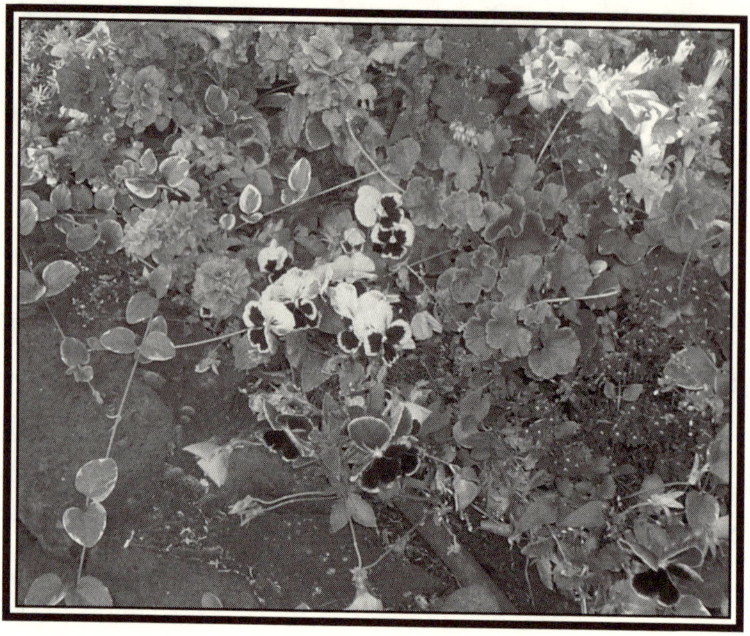

A Trip to Town

LET yourself now go to that other place, the one that feels good. As you go there, you can allow yourself to relax. It can be very comfortable, as if you were being carried on gossamer wings. I wonder where the word *gossamer* came from. It feels nice. Continue to relax even more, and you may see things float before your eyes. You may hear soft sounds in the distance. These sounds can relax you even more, shifting you quickly to that other space. You may find you are in more places than you realize. One of the things that you may see is a ledger book. Ledger books have credits on one side and debits on the other side. Some of these debits and credits are balanced, and some are not. If you look closely, you may see that some debts are long standing. Sometimes an auditor will come in and look at these ledgers and he will often say, "Now the debts have been paid and the books are cleared and balanced." Many other things are now balanced. What a relief!

Drift down as if you were a leaf falling from a tree, floating gently down into the land of the stories. This story begins with a lovely woman in her garden. She is working and planting, transplanting, feeding, and doing all those things that gardeners do. She loves this. It is very obvious, for her garden shows it. The plants are healthy, the flowers are brilliant colors. It is as if the flowers bow to her with respect and love, and she bows back to them. The soil feels rich under her fingers. Often she takes some beautiful flowers and gives them to people. Because she cares so much about her garden, they are replaced very quickly with other beautiful blooms. This day, she has gathered a bunch of them in her basket. She begins walking on the road to town, feeling the breeze, looking at the blue sky as she walks. She sends love to everything she sets her eyes on. As she walks, she thinks about another time in the distant past. It was a time when she was taking care of her younger brother, for that is what he needed at that time. He was preparing for a race. Every day she helped him prepare, helping him improve his technique, running beside him, taking care of him in the way she knew best. She helped him win. She smiled as she thought, "Now he has grown up and can take care of himself and it's my time now." She feels very rich. As she passes people on the way to town, it is obvious how they honor her. She is well loved and respected. Everyone she meets honors her for who she is. She feels very blessed because she has many people taking care of her and her heart is full. She passes out her lovely flowers to her dear friends. Even the animals seem to honor her. They know that she is filled with such love, and even *they* wish to take care of her. It is not that she does anything extraordinary. She is honored simply for who she is. She loves to go into town to do her shopping because by the time she gets around her town, her flowers have been all been given out, so she has room for her purchases. The shop people love to have her in their shops. She has a great deal of fun laughing and joking while she does her shopping, chatting about her garden, for she has not only flowers, but tasty vegetables in her garden. She passes on the secrets that she has learned, and sometimes she gives vegetables away as well. This day she has a grand and glorious time, and visits new stores that weren't there the last time she was in town, exploring because she enjoys everything she does. She has her share of problems like everyone else, but she encounters them, then steps over, around, or through them and keeps going. The owner of the new shop has already heard about her and is pleased to have her in his shop. Like all stores that have grand opening specials, he gives her a gift as a token of his respect and caring, and feels very blessed. She finishes her shopping and prepares to walk home. Her heart feels full, and she gives hugs and receives them, makes plans to see some of her friends socially, and takes with her, some of the things that she has been given by the other people. She thinks of these beautiful people and their sharing. Then she smiles inside for she knows she is like that also. She knows that she could never be alone in her life, for there are so many wonderful people who give to her as she gives to them, with ease, with love, and with joy. She pats her basket as she walks home, for she has some new seeds that she is going to plant in her garden. She is excited because she can't wait to see what they turn out to be.

How easy it is to give up control and go on automatic pilot. Because, when you try to guide the boat, you hang on too tightly, and it doesn't go where you want it to go. Sometimes it is better to take your hand off the controls and let the boat go on its own. Sometimes it will go in the same direction, and sometimes it changes directions. And sometimes it is a big relief not to hold on too tightly. By the way, the gossamer wings can take you to new places where your heart soars and the knowledge comes pouring in like beautiful sparkling raindrops. It can be exhilarating.

Feel yourself float on the currents of the wind. Sometimes the currents have a certain familiar smell.

When I was a little girl we had radio, and I would often use it as background noise. Sometimes the background was irritating and sometimes it was soothing, occasionally it was funny, very comforting. It had all those qualities. Now that I am grown up, it is nice to know that I can turn the dial to whatever I want, and tune into whatever station I want, at whatever volume I want so that I can either focus on it very loudly, or have it run softly through the background. Now, turn your station to the one you want, for now there are many more stations than there were before. Some of these signals come from far-away places. How nice it is that they go right down to the ground. Now you can, if you want, search around and find one of those signals and ride it back down here to the ground.

Afterword

FROM ancient times, people gathered near the campfire to listen to tales told by the story tellers. Under a starry canopy or inside a shelter, the surroundings melted into the darkness, the flames flickered and formed evocative shapes as day-to-day life dissipated and the story became real, capturing the listeners' imagination.

Actual events would be told as stories, thus keeping a historical record orally before writing existed. These events were told to others in the community, a kind of verbal newspaper. The images kept the members of the tribe interested, informed so they felt part of the group. The stories would also be made into songs that both informed and entertained.

The history of the tribe was passed along to the new generations in the form of stories, which made it easier to remember. In the telling, the listener would get images, feelings or sounds in his head which allowed him to be a distant participant in the story. In addition to reporting actual events, stories were used as teaching tools, illustrating a point the teller wanted to make. Other stories would emphasize natural emotions and then give a variety of examples of how to deal with these intense feelings. When writing was invented, the stories took a written form in addition to the oral tradition.

Story tellers throughout history were important in all cultures, and people listened eagerly. Musicians made the stories into songs, and writers made them into plays. A good story teller made it seem as if the listener were there in the story as the teller either gave vivid and detailed images, or told the tale in such a way that the listener made his own images. "Fantasy, imagination, stream of consciousness, day dreaming, imagery, visualization, guided imagery, waking dreams, reverie, active imagination are all words that have been used to describe imagery."... "Primitive man did not need to be aware of visualization; it was the way in which he related to the world." "[1]

The field of psychology has given much attention and research to the power of visualization or imagery. A fact that often has been overlooked is that stories can affect change, dramatic or subtle. Whether through fairy tales, metaphors, hypnosis or imagery techniques, the human brain makes associations relevant to the person's situation. In his book, *Personal Mythology*[2], David Feinstein talks about writing your own Fairy Tale, your personal myth.

---

1 Carlson Collins, M.J. *All Paths Lead to the Mountain Top.* Doctoral Dissertation. San Raphael, CA: Columbia Pacific University, 1986.

2 Feinstein, Ph.D., David & Krippner, Ph.D. Stanley. *Personal Mythology.* Los Angeles: Jeremy P. Tarcher, Inc. ,1988

Much has been studied and written about the mind-body connection and the power of images and imagination to effect change. Those who knew Milton Erikson marveled at his ability to produce profound changes in a person with a short conversation in which he would tell a story that appeared to have no relation to the problem the person had. Many studied Milton Erikson, including Ernest Rossi who wrote *The Psychobiology of Mind-Body Healing: New Concepts of Therapeutic Hypnosis*[3].

Joseph Campbell, a well known mythologist, studied myths and tales from around the world.[4] His work has been archived and expanded by Jonathan Young.

"Imagery in healing is probably best known for its direct effects on physiology," according to Martin Rossman, M.D., and David Bressler, Ph.D founders of the Academy for Guided Imagery. "Through imagery you can stimulate changes in many body functions usually considered inaccessible to conscious influence."[5] It seems amazing that the images the imagination produces can actually affect people physically.

3 Rossi, Ernest Lawrence. *The Psychobiology of Mind-Body Healing: New Concepts of Therapeutic Hypnosis.* New York: W.W. Norton & Company, Inc., 1983, revised 1993.

4 Campbell, Joseph, *The Hero with a Thousand Faces.* Bollinger Series XVII: 1949.

5 Rossman, M.D., Martin, and Bressler, PhD., David. From www.healthyroads.com.

In addition to stories and imagery affecting the physical body, the emotional state can be greatly affected also. Stories can initiate strong emotions or help release them. Every strong emotion causes chemical changes in the body so transformation of harmful emotions can be helpful.

The stories in this book were created almost automatically. A client would arrive with a problem and then images would start in my head—either pictures or words. Sometimes a full story would emerge. Other times, there were metaphor images, which I would deliberately put together to make a story, or simply a series of images to make the same point.

I would like to thank Carol Quinn for her substantial input in the Meditations Section of the book.

The first such story that I created was in response to a problem a three-year-old boy had. He had to have an operation to put a tube in his head to drain excess fluid. This tube came from his head and ran under his skin down to his abdomen where the fluid drained. After the operation, he kept pulling at the tube. I asked myself how I could help him accept the presence of the tube, since it was to be permanent. Thus *The Critter* story was born. After I first told him the story, he asked for it two more times and then he no longer pulled at his tube. Even though this story was designed for a three year old, it can apply to anyone—children or adults who need to accept something they don't want to accept, whether it is a hip replacement, pins to hold a broken bone in place, or a person that they need to care for moving into their home. Acceptance is the key word for this story.

These stories are designed for specific results but our minds are so creative and multi-dimensional that we make connections that could not be done consciously. It is helpful to become open to new ideas, attitudes and experiences. Sometimes we get stuck in old viewpoints or actions, and stories and images can help us to accept change so that we can move forward in a balanced healthy way. We can be inspired to strengthen our values and live the best life we can.

These stories are catalytic in helping transform the perspective of readers and listeners to spur them to action or help them relax into balance and the natural rhythm of life.

Simply, Transformational Tales.

Colophon
Typeset in Warnock Pro and Myriad Pro
Cover Design by Douglas E. Thompson
Cover illustration: Rainbow over ocean © Murat Verdiesen
Printed by BookMasters, Inc., Ashland, Ohio